HEALING POWER OF HERBS

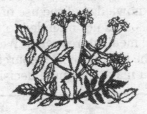

Dr. John Heinerman

◆◆◆

Cover Photo by Michael Skott

NOTE: *The Healing Power of Herbs* is intended to broaden your knowledge of the use of herbs for medicinal purposes. It is not intended to take the place of conventional medical treatment. We strongly urge that you seek the best medical resources available to you to help you make informed decisions.

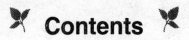

Contents

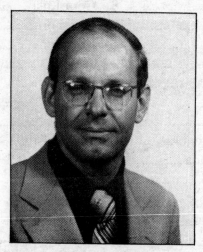

John Heinerman, Ph.D., a medical anthropologist and author of more than a dozen books, has researched herbs and their medicinal properties all over the world, working with folk healers and scientists as well as medical doctors. He lives and works in Salt Lake City, Utah.

Introduction

Throughout our history, we have relied on herbs for many reasons. We have used them to soothe our pain and heal our wounds. We have ingested them to feel better and rubbed them on our bodies to, hopefully, look better. We have relied on them to flavor our foods — and to hide the unmistakeable odor of them going 'off'.

In this book distinguished medical anthropologist and researcher Dr. John Heinerman spotlights 50 of the most popular, and useful, herbs of all time. Many of them contain a broad range of health enhancing properties although each generally has a particular value in the treatment of a specific ailment. In his travels, Heinerman has talked directly to many people whose health has been dramatically helped by herbs and he recounts some of these case histories in the following pages.

Herbs work well in several different forms. The most convenient and preferred method to take them today is in the form of gelatin capsules. But they are also efficient in teas and fluid extracts. On pp. 92-93, you will discover how to make these teas and extracts.

On pp. 94-97, there is a handy cross reference that lists ailments and the herbs that can help.

While many herbs are forms of food which can improve your health because of their vitamin and mineral content, others work, more accurately, as natural drugs. Here, Dr. Heinerman presents only those herbs which, in his experience and research, will do the most good, with the least amount of discomfort. In cases where a potential problem is likely to arise, he has carefully noted the steps to be taken.

Alfalfa

The king of herbs!

Many centuries ago, the Arabs discovered, quite by accident, that when their weaker horses and camels had a chance to graze on this common field grass, they ran faster and were stronger than grain-fed animals. For this reason, they named it alfalfa.

The name itself is comprised of two parts: **AL** from Allah, in honor of their God, and **FALF**, which meant 'Father of All Foods!'

Alfalfa holds the distinction of being a combination food plant/medicine plant. Just think of being able to eat a piece of cake that will make you healthier! That's pretty much the case here — you get food and medicine in one herb. In fact, there's alfalfa in a capsule. Or a warm cup of tea.

Granted, the latter may taste a little like a cup of freshly brewed hay — that's what it is. But you can't knock something just because the aroma may remind you of breakfast for a dairy herd. In fact the statistics on alfalfa are nothing short of amazing. Two tablespoonfuls, or about 10 capsules, contains:

- Twice as much calcium as an ordinary glass of milk
- Almost as much protein as one fried hamburger
- Nearly the same amount of iron as two ounces of liver
- Enough B-complex for the most jangled nerves
- Plenty of enzymes for good metabolism of ingested fats
- Sufficient fiber to lower the highest cholesterol

When it comes to nourishment and healing it truly is, as one of my folksy herbalist colleagues has aptly described it, 'the Big Daddy of 'em all!'

A true story of a serious infection that would have turned

gangrenous but for alfalfa was related by the late Henry G. Bieler, M.D., once the personal physician to movie stars like Gloria Swanson and Gary Cooper, in his book, *Food is Your Best Medicine:*

> I traveled across the sagebrush for nearly a hundred miles to see a farmer who had suffered a discharging leg ulcer for several years. The whole right leg was greatly swollen and a foul crater was located just above the ankle.
>
> I had to get into him ... [some] alkaline vegetable juices of various types. But it was late fall and no vegetables were growing. Nor were there any supermarkets with daily supplies of fresh vegetables from distant farms. The only medically useful plant growing on the farm at that time of year was alfalfa.
>
> "We'll feed him alfalfa," I said. His wife looked flabbergasted ...

> The crusty old farmer protested that only his cows ate stuff like that, and he insisted he was NO cow! But in the end he was persuaded to drink the alfalfa tea his wife made for him every couple of hours. According to Dr. Bieler, "In time ... the ulcer healed entirely and the swelling disappeared."

For problems of this type, four cups of alfalfa tea a day is the recommended dosage. Or, if you prefer, you can take 12 capsules, four three times a day with meals.

This herb is a marvelous remedy for disorders of the bones, particularly fractures, osteoporosis and, especially, arthritis. It provides a tremendous amount of calcium as well as potassium and phosphorus, and significant anti-inflammatory elements including copper and zinc.

If you're crippled with any of the foregoing problems, you ought to be using alfalfa in a big way! I don't recommend it in the fluid extract form, because the alcohol will destroy many of its life-giving vitamins and enzymes. It's best to use it in tea or capsule form only.

Aloe Vera

Lasting comfort

Among the three dozen books on health, nutrition, and herbal folk medicine that I've written in the last 15 years, there was one I published a decade ago simply called *Aloe Vera, Jojoba and Yucca*. In it, I showed how magnificently aloe vera helped to heal skin which had been damaged by radiation, fire, or caustic or boiling materials.

For less severe problems, like bedsores and hemorrhoids, it's the perfect medication. Where else, pray tell, are you going to get so much simple relief from pain than from a little application of the natural gel that oozes out of any cut aloe vera leaf?

A sweet little old lady named Marjorie Knutsen, who actually was, believe it or not, from Pasadena, California, wrote me awhile back, claiming she had suffered from irritable bowel syndrome — which plagues millions of people — for many years and hadn't had much help from routine therapy. Someone told her that aloe vera leaf and cascara sagrada bark (see pp. 19-20) work well together for intestinal tract disorders. So she took a combination of both — three capsules each, twice daily on an empty stomach, with a full glass of water — for 10 days and discovered to her amazement that her problem was clearing up.

When she fully recovered, she told a friend, who was suffering from colitis. And guess what? That friend started using the same combination, and in no time at all, she, too, felt greatly improved. Of course, as Marjorie herself explained, "People need to see their doctors, too, about conditions like this!"

Bayberry

Sore throat remedy

Its other name is wax myrtle, but we know this herb best as bayberry. It is an evergreen shrub or tree which can grow, in some cases, as tall as 35 feet. Sometimes, they are used as Christmas trees.

Some years ago, in 1983, I spent Christmas Eve with a friend of mine, a delightful fellow named Tom Smith, in Palestine, Texas. Tom had planned to be Father Christmas — Santa Claus — that night to delight his five children and 'surprise' his wife with a big bag of gifts. But when I arrived, Tom was in his suit but didn't feel at all up to the task at hand. He was suffering the miseries of a raging sore throat.

I looked around the house, spotted the decorated tree in the corner — a bayberry — and said: "Tom, I think I have just the thing for you. Trust me, I can clip a few of these grayish green twigs off that tree and make some tea for you." So I made the tea and instructed him to gargle, then swallow, the concoction.

So there he sat on a kitchen chair, all decked out in his red and white suit and the little red Santa hat, with his head tilted back, making strange noises every few seconds or so. He wasn't too impressed with my prescription. "This stuff tastes gosh-awful!" he protested. Then he went back to his gargling. But, happily, in less than half an hour, the inflammation in Tom's throat had subsided enough for him to make his grand entrance complete with heavy bag and a pretty good, "Ho! Ho! Ho!"

Four capsules taken with warm water twice daily, or 12 drops of fluid extract twice daily in the back of the throat, should also work. I always use the tea and I personally think it is best by far in treating this particular kind of problem.

Black Cohosh

Every woman's botanical friend

In the 19th century, herbs were utilized a lot more by the medical profession than they are at present. Sometimes by consulting a few of the old medical reference works published back then we are better able to understand, from a clinical perspective, the therapeutic benefits and limitations of particular plants.

One such authority now frequently consulted is John V. Shoemaker, M.D. His *Practical Treatise on Materia Medica & Therapeutica* (Rev. 7th Ed.) was a standard textbook for many medical students in the eastern United States from 1889 to 1910. For over 31 years, Dr. Shoemaker was a Professor of Clinical Medicine at the Medico-Chirurgical College in Philadelphia, where several thousand aspiring doctors benefitted from his lectures.

Dr. Shoemaker had many good things to say about black cohosh: "The menstrual flow is increased, and some aphrodisiac qualities have been ascribed to (it)." Furthermore, " ... it is beneficial in melancholia, especially when that condition is associated with functional or organic uterine or ovarian disorder." It had also been "found useful in rheumatoid arthritis" in women, he asserted.

"The fluid extract is the best and most reliable preparation for this," he wrote.

Between 10-15 drops under the tongue is suggested. But I'm inclined to think that capsules (3-4 daily) would work just as well.

He also declared that it was excellent for difficult and painful menstruation (dysmenorrhea), excessively prolonged menstruation (menorrhagia), and irregular bleeding from the uterus between periods (metrorrhagia), but warned against pregnant women using it other than just before their actual delivery time.

Black Walnut

Montezuma's revenge

Because of my own interest in the early history of ancient Mesoamerica (Mexico and Central America combined) and my professional background in anthropology, I've joined fellow scientists from time to time on various archaeological digs in and around the Yucatan Peninsula.

Living conditions there aren't always the greatest. If the hungry ticks with their built-in heat sensors that drop from the trees onto your neck don't get you first, then the terrible heat and stifling humidity of the torrid jungle most certainly will.

But the water is what saps your strength the most. Those little invisible microbes with the big, long Latin names can quickly reduce the mightiest Olympian warrior to panty-waist puniness in no time at all. Put another way: After drinking from the local supply, it feels as though a big Mack truck just collided with your entire gastrointestinal tract. No wonder they calls this 'Montezuma's revenge!'

Early on in my expeditions, I learned what to take with me to avoid similar miseries. The very best thing, I discovered, was black walnut capsules. I'd take four of them every time I suspected the safety of the water I was drinking. And while the rest of my buddies were running or, in some cases, almost crawling or staggering to the nearest bushes, desperately clutching their bellies, I tried to refrain from laughing. But, I'll have to admit now, that not making a clever comment was just about the hardest temptation I believe I ever had to cope with in my life!

Blessed Thistle

Nourishment for nursing moms

This member of the daisy family is closely allied to other thistles. As such, it has physical characteristics which make it more repugnant than desirable. For one thing, the leaves are very spiny and spear-pointed. For another, the bitterness comes quite high on the list of truly yucky-tasting herbs. But in spite of these objectionable aspects it does have powerful redeeming qualities.

Chief among these powers is its ability to help nursing moms have plenty of milk when breast-feeding their infants. It seems that it's the bitter alkaloid called *cnicin* which irritates the mammary glands just enough so that they secrete more milk than might ordinarily be the case.

Because of the high calcium and iron contents in blessed thistle, moms who take it regularly yield a richer and superior milk supply than those who don't.

Almost 60 years ago, it was common for many women in Great Britain to rely upon this herb to ensure adequate daily supplies of milk for their babies.

Moms would drink 1 cup of warm tea about 30 minutes before feeding time began. Or they might take some herbal pills (4 capsules today) with a glass of warm water. However, the fluid extract didn't seem to have much of an effect this way. It appears from the evidence at hand, that moderate heat in the form of warm liquid of some kind is the key to making this herb work the best.

Buchu

For kidneys, bladder and prostate

We all owe a debt of gratitude to the primitive Hottentot tribesmen of southern Africa for introducing the healing miracles of buchu leaf to the rest of the world. The Hottentots had been using this aromatic shrub for just about every ailment imaginable for thousands of years before contact was ever first made with European explorers, probably sometime in the early 17th century.

As men and women become older, bladder problems become much frequent. Buchu is the native remedy used to treat this type of infirmity.

An early Dutch herbalist named Pappe furnished us with the first detailed account of the native African uses and methods of application for buchu during the early 19th century in his book, *Florae Capensis Medicae Prodromus*, which appeared in Capetown in 1857. Pappe made a special note that the leaf was almost always used by the Hottentots mixed with some kind of alcohol or vinegar. The judicious use of fermented or sour beverages of some type appeared to be important in the effective use of the buchu. Ordinary water, it seemed, simply did not have the same effect.

A tea was usually made by simmering some of the buchu leaves in brandy or vinegar and then drinking it when it was sufficiently cooled. Usually 2 cups regularly every day was sufficient to beat most infections of the kidneys, bladder and prostate but the dosage was increased if the condition was serious — and the symptoms were not alleviated by the usual dose.

When using a fluid extract of buchu, figure on taking about 15 drops beneath the tongue three times a day. Capsules (5 daily) may also be used, but take these with a little apple ci-

15

der vinegar or brandy instead of water.

A lot of older men today suffer from prostate problems, especially inflammation. The most common symptoms include feeling off color, shivery chills, a temperature that escalates to fever level, flu-like aches and pains all over the body, but especially so in the back, a heavy feeling between the legs in the groin area, discomfort on sitting down or urinating and agonizing bowel movements.

According to Pappe, the Hottentots just gave large amounts of their slightly alcoholic or fermented leaf brew to their older warriors who suffered from the same problem. In virtually no time at all these guys were up and around, busy as ever. Apparently several camphor-like compounds within the leaf, which accounts for the aromatic odor, are the key to reversing inflammation and infection of the prostate.

This wonderful Hottentot folk remedy has also great value for women. It is very effective in clearing up infections of the urethra and vagina.

About the same amounts of tea, fluid extract and capsules cited for bladder disorders should be followed for prostate difficulties. Buchu also happens to be of very high value in treating kidney stones and urinary tract infection. For the latter condition, I suggest a combination of cranberry in capsule form (3 capsules) and buchu (2 capsules) together. Or take a ½ cup of each tea or a dozen drops of each fluid extract beneath the tongue.

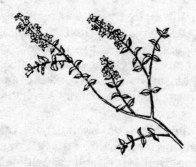

Butcher's Broom

Sweeps away poisons

T he matured branches of this herb used to be bound into bundles and sold to butchers in old England for sweeping their cutting blocks clean — hence the name. One British herbalist of a few centuries ago observed that butcher's broom was used to preserve 'hanged meat' from being eaten by mice.

Like Paris and other of the great European capitals, London has its share of gypsies. They are well regarded for their great knowledge of natural remedies and I spent some time talking with one of their herbalists during a 1980 visit to England. He was very enthusiastic about butcher's broom. He said that broom flowers were an excellent cure for yellow jaundice and that the bramble tops and broom tops, together, were a very old West Country — specifically the county of Dorset — remedy for all kinds of kidney complaints. I had to struggle with his accent sometimes but I understood well enough when he told me that it would: "... heal them that's pretty far gone, too, what no drabengo (doctor) couldn't cure for ever so, give'n what medicine he would."

Three capsules, or 1 cup of tea or 15 drops of the fluid extract is recommended for cleaning out the liver or kidneys.

Butcher's broom is widely used in many rural areas of Europe. To hear the shepherds in the mountainous province of Auvergne in south-central France tell it, for example, this herb is the best thing known to build up body resistance against viper bites. French scientists studying the main component of broom tops, called *spartein*, have discovered that it detoxifies snake venom. The complex protein structure which comprises such deadly poison is broken up in the presence of spartein.

The mountain shepherds sometimes drink a half cup of the tea each day for several months at a time to build up their immunity against such bites. I have no doubt that a regular daily dosage of 3 to 5 capsules of broom would provide significant protection against the bite of a rattlesnake, for instance.

But there are apparently other uses for the broom's power in sweeping poisons out of the system. On another of my many travels, I had occasion to go through Heathrow Airport in London on my way to Ethiopia and mainland China with the American Medical Students Association. During our brief layover there, I chanced to meet up with a British 'bobby', as they're called, or local street cop and he was absolutely fascinated about my involvement in herbal and folk medicine research. He was a big fan of natural medicine of all kinds, and he told me this story about butcher's broom.

He said that from childhood he had periodically suffered from bronchial asthma, especially in the winter time when the air was damp and the fog, for which London is legendary, was inescapable.

He recounted how he took some butcher's broom capsules — the dosage he used was 5 capsules — with some black- or green-leaf tea whenever he had an attack of belabored breathing. He claimed that the combination of the two enabled him to almost immediately inhale and exhale a lot better.

He said that when he first took the capsules, he drank them down with ordinary cool or cold water and that "nothing really happened." But when he took them with the warm or hot tea "it really opened me up something grand," he said. I had not heard of this before but I recommend anyone who experiences difficulty breathing as the result of colds or bronchitis to try the policeman's remedy.

Cascara Sagrada

Nature's colon cleanser

Some health-food purists and finicky herbalists like to insist that if an herb isn't absolutely fresh, then it isn't any good. Well, I'd like to take exception to that philosophy. In certain instances if it is fresh it will probably make you as sick as a dog!

That is certainly true of cascara sagrada. Consider this little lesson in botanical medicine: When the reddish-brown bark is removed from trees with trunk diameters measuring 10 centimeters or more, it must be stored in large warehouses for about a year before it can be used.

And what if it isn't? Well, if you were to use the fresh bark straight from the tree, either as a tea or encapsulated powder, you would most likely be throwing up very soon. That is because the fresh bark has powerful emetic principles which can only be made friendly through long-term drying and aging.

One naturopathic physician I know in Vancouver, Canada, swears by this bark and has a stack of patient's testimonials demonstrating its marvelous and quick-acting effectiveness. "Dr. Heinerman," he told me one day when I was in his office, "there is nothing — and I mean nothing — that comes close to curing constipation like this little number." At the same time he held up a bottle of capsules containing this herb.

"Really works that well?" I queried.

"Better than that," he rejoined with positiveness.

He then proceeded to explain that not only does it evoke bowel movements, but it also actually "gives shape and substance to the evacuated wastes. Those of my patients with difficult bowel movements don't find any more hard marbles or messy diarrhea to contend with after being on cascara for a while," he added.

"What is the dosage you recommend and which form works the best?" I asked with a professional interest of my own.

"First of all, I think the capsules work the quickest. The tea is okay, but not as quick or easy as the capsules." I advise my patients to take 3 capsules on an empty stomach with some mineral or seltzer water. If neither of them are available, then I recommend a little 7-Up, perhaps.

"The combination of the two seems to work better than when taken with ordinary water. Sometimes a few of my more difficult cases must repeat this amount four hours later, but not very often."

My naturopathic friend thought that a cup of the warm tea in between meals ought to have the desired effect.

"The thing to remember about this herb," he stated, "is that it's sort of like a liquid Drano or Mr. Plumber on your colon. It really seems to get things cleaned out pretty thoroughly with minimal effort. I prefer it over other laxatives by far."

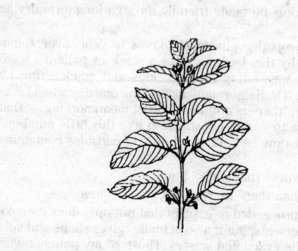

Catnip

Say good-bye to colds and flu

The same stuff in catnip that makes felines go absolutely bonkers also lowers fevers, dries up post-nasal drip, gets rid of sledgehammer headaches and relieves sore aching bones due to colds and flus. The active compound we're speaking about here has been designated as *cis-trans-nepetalactone*.

An old Norwegian woman from one of the small Mormon communities in south-central Utah recalled how her own mother used to doctor her and all of her brothers and sisters with this herb when they were young. "Every ache and pain associated with childhood diseases or the miseries of influenza was successfully met with this little herb," she asserted. "No one was ever sick when they took their catnip every day."

Besides as tea (2-3 warm cups daily), catnip may also be taken in gelatin capsules (4 twice or thrice daily on an empty stomach) or fluid extract (20 drops beneath the tongue once or twice daily as needed). The key here seems to be taking the herb with something warm. This *nepetalactone* exercises a strong stimulating effect on the brain's *endorphins*, which help to relieve pain, and on the white blood cells of the immune system which destroy harmful viruses.

It is interesting to note that catnip's *nepetalactone* is somewhat similar in its chemical structure to the sedative *valepotriates* in valerian, which gives the plant its infamous 'dirty socks' smell.

Cayenne Pepper
Stops the bleeding

My own experiences with *capsicum* go back to 1977 and my first archaeological dig in the Yucatan Peninsula of southeastern Mexico. One of our interpreters — a guy named Hernando Antonio de Maria y Sanchez (we called him 'Harry') — would sit in the shade during break-time and dip peeled sour orange sections in a little bit of cayenne powder. He and his colleagues swore by this as an aid to health and long life.

And there certainly seems to be a biochemical synergism of some kind between the fiery properties of *capsaicin* in the red pepper and the antibacterial ascorbic acid in citrus fruits. I recommend 3 capsules of cayenne pepper with a glass of freshly squeezed orange juice as a terrific cold fighter.

But the most remarkable actions of capsicum appear to be with the circulating blood plasma. Internally, it can reduce platelet stickiness so that clots don't form. Used externally, it works wonders in stopping bleeding.

Some years ago eating lunch with a Registered Nurse here in Utah, I accidentally cut through the skin webbing between my right thumb and forefinger. While my nurse friend was still wondering what to do, I walked to the serving window and asked for some cayenne pepper.

I piled generous amounts of cayenne on the cut. Within a couple of minutes, ALL bleeding had ceased entirely, though the top and surrounding area looked worse than it was.

My companion asked where I learned about this. I told her about a colleague on one of my expeditions who cut himself while clearing jungle undergrowth — and how we had watched in fascination as he applied cayenne, immediately staunching the wound.

Chamomile

For a good night's sleep

The most interesting group of compounds in both species of chamomile (Roman and German) are the *azulenes*. They give the extracted oil a deep ink-blue color and there is a slight rubbery tone to the odor. There are different types of azulenes: *chamazulene, prochamazulene, guaiazulene* and others.

These are noted for their anti-allergenic and anti-inflammatory properties. They prevent the discharge of histamine in the body, which triggers allergic reactions — like sneezing — for instance, or the sensations of pain. But one of the primary functions appears to be as a muscle-relaxant.

A report in *Food & Cosmetics Toxicology* (15:173-81, 1977), emphasized how well these azulene compounds stimulate liver regeneration in rats which had had portions of that organ surgically removed. So 3 capsules of chamomile with a glass of low-sodium V-8 or tomato juice (which also regenerates the liver), along with 2 capsules of dandelion root each day, will do wonders for that organ.

I believe I was among the first to pinpoint the source of this remarkable sedative property as being the amino acid, *tryptophan*, in my book, *The Science of Herbal Medicine*. My initial research was later cited by chemists Connie Mann and E. John Staba of the College of Pharmacy at the University of Minnesota in Minneapolis, in Volume One of *Herbs, Spices, and Medicinal Plants: Recent Advances in Botany, Horticulture, and Pharmacology*. Tryptophan is the 'tune' which chamomile 'sings' to restless nerves and agitated brains.

A cup of warm tea or 4 capsules taken with some warm water should give you a good night's sleep.

Chaparral

Victory over cancer

The desert chaparral, or creosote bush, occupies one of the most important places in the healing arts, particularly in the prevention and treatment of cancer. This plant probably is one of the most potent chemotherapeutic weapons to be found in nature, together with goldenseal root and red clover blossoms.

Of all the herbs, I favor the aforementioned three the best. And of that trio, chaparral sits tall in the saddle in the ride to recovery for those who've been stricken with the dreaded 'Big C'.

With unparalleled ingenuity, this shrub has managed to overcome, with pit-bull determination, the challenge of a fiercely hostile environment. Against animal assailants, including just about all insects imaginable, its repellent odor and taste serve as protection and cause its avoidance by all except, now and then, a starving jackrabbit or a nest-building pack rat.

As for the supreme desert enemy of all, this pliant plant can outride even the most forbidding drought. It favors the meanest clay, the driest sand, and hardpan that is almost concrete-firm. Even in bleak Death Valley, California, you will find chaparral — even though not much of anything else can grow there!

Let me say a few words about chaparral's incredibly strong anti-growth substance. It is called NDGA, an abbreviation for a naturally-occurring chemical called *nordihydroguaiaretic acid*. The September 2nd, 1972, issue of *Chemistry and Industry* reported that "NDGA has been shown to be one of the most effective anti-oxidants known."

What this means, for one thing, is that it shoots down bad guy microbes like salmonella, Candida yeast and other assorted pathogens. At another level, it destroys the 'sharks' called *free radicals* that zip madly through the cells of our bodies and rip and tear at our molecules. Scientists have now concluded that there is a definite connection between these mad molecules with their crazily-spinning electrons and such ailments as arthritis, cancer and coronary disease — as well as many of the other accompanying effects of the aging process. As an antioxidant, NDGA effectively degrades, neutralizes, and detoxifies the free radicals inside each of us. It is a very powerful agent in fighting the ravages of AIDS as well.

Back in 1969-70, chaparral made numerous headlines and evening newscasts in papers and on radio and TV all over the West. One, in particular, that I liked above the rest, was this from an Arizona newspaper article: "Is Chaparral The Medical Miracle Doctors Have Been Looking For?"

The Case of Ernest Farr

An 87-year-old Mormon temple worker, Ernest Farr, living in Mesa, Arizona, had undergone three operations to remove a malignant facial lesion, but the growth returned each time in larger form. Farr became weak and pale and lost considerable weight.

As the November, 1970 edition of the *Rocky Mountain Medical Journal* recounted, "A wedge biopsy of the facial lesion and a needle biopsy of the neck mass revealed malignant melanoma.

"His attending physicians recommended surgical excision ... with a radical neck dissection. But Mr. Farr decided against any further treatment. He told one of his daughters: 'I've suffered enough at their hands already, and I intend to go back home and die in dignity.'"

He began brewing up large potfuls of this old Indian remedy traditionally used for colds, rheumatism, venereal disease, bowel cramps, gout and arthritis. He made chaparral tea by steeping the dried leaves and stems (2 small handfuls) in hot water (1 quart). He simmered the tea on low heat for seven minutes and then removed it from the stove and let it steep, covered, for up to 12 hours! This is a very important key to making chaparral tea that works! He took no other medication.

The story of his remarkable recovery was recounted in an interview — it was tape recorded and preserved — that he gave in 1970. Both a copy of the tape and the typed transcript were supplied to me by Kay Windes of Mesa, to whom I extend my grateful thanks. Here are Mr. Farr's own words from that tape:

"After I had been back here in Mesa a few weeks, my daughter called up long distance and said, 'Dad, how are you feeling?' I said, 'Well, I am feeling ever so much better. My face is all healed up ... The lump on my face has gone down. The incision is healed and I am feeling ever so much better.'

"The next day Dr. (C.R.) Smart (the attending physician in Salt Lake City) called up my daughter and asked, 'How is your father? Is he still alive?' And she (responded), 'I just talked to him yesterday and he said his face was all cleared and he was feeling so much better.'

"The doctor could not believe her and said, 'I have to see this for myself.' So the doctor sent for me to come back to Salt Lake. When he saw my face, it was all healed up. First thing he done, he got a camera and took about 13 pictures ... he was so surprised, and he said, 'Now, Mr. Farr, I want you to be here at 7:00 tomorrow morning'.

"The next morning he took me into a room where they have a group for consultations and all the doctors and staff were there and he had me tell them all about this wonderful chaparral. I told them about the people I knew that had been cured by it, both of cancer and of arthritis."

Mr. Farr agreed to send the doctors plenty of chaparral with instructions on how to make the tea for their terminally-ill patients. According to what two of the doctors told him later on by phone, " ... for many of them, they are responding very nicely to it."

A dosage of 4 cups of chaparral tea, or 8 capsules three times a day, or 15 drops of fluid extract four times daily on an empty stomach is recommended.

Chickweed

Laundering dirty blood

Ask just about any farmer what he thinks of chickweed, and he's liable to utter a stream of profane epithets that are certainly beyond 'gosh-darned' and 'golly gee-whiz' by a mile or more. For, you see, chickweed is the herb that farmers love to curse and swear at along with prickly tumbleweeds, milk weeds, couch grass and other obnoxious plants.

But while many may malign weeds through ignorance and prejudice, others who are more enlightened on the subject give the lowly chickweed some of the dignity it truly deserves. This is undoubtedly what I had in mind some years ago, when a nosy TV reporter shoved a microphone into my face and flippantly asked me: "Doctor Heinerman, just what is it that you do?" Not missing a beat, I replied dead pan: "Why, I give respect to weeds!"

And this is precisely how I feel about chickweed. Forget about its unbecoming ways, and realize for a moment just how much of a tonic value it can have for tired blood. When you think about it, this herb seems to be just the thing for cleaning up dirty blood. If you've been on a junk food binge or have been practicing careless eating habits — then have I got an herb for you!

Two cups a day, 6 capsules or 20 drops under the tongue is not only going to redeem your blood from purgatory pollution. But it's also apt to have it shouting, "Glory! Hallelujah!" if you keep taking it long enough.

Cranberry

For urinary tract infection

Women are more prone to urinary tract infections than men because the female urethra is shorter, and the bladder is thus closer to sources of bacterial contamination. Women can cut down the chances of getting UTIs by avoiding tight pantyhose, nylon underpants without a cotton crotch, and skin-tight jeans. Keeping the vaginal area very clean is also important. Wipe only from front to back after every bowel movement. It also makes sense for a woman to empty her bladder after having had sexual intercourse.

UTIs can develop into serious and even life-threatening infections of the kidneys. These disorders are treatable and even preventable. Recent medical research has demonstrated the powers of cranberry juice, preferably as an encapsulated powder, for treating this condition.

Those of us who've celebrated Thanksgiving in style know that such a feast wouldn't be complete without the customary turkey and cranberry sauce. Well, the powdered juice of fresh cranberries is a medical marvel.

Dr. A.E. Sobota of Youngstown State University in Youngstown, Ohio, had much to say about it in the May, 1984, issue of *The Journal of Urology.* He claims that he has identified a special factor in the juice that seems to make pathogenic (disease-carrying) bacteria less likely to cling to the surface of bladder and urinary tract cells. He isn't quite sure what the mystery substance responsible for this anti-cling action is, but he says the factor shows up in animal and human urine within one to three hours after taking cranberry juice and may stay potent for up to 15 hours.

His study was preceded by one which appeared in the September, 1967, *Journal of the American Dietetic Associa-*

tion, in which a group of doctors from the V.A. Hospital in the Bronx, New York, tested cranberry juice on some male patients and discovered that it was excellent therapy for UTIs as well as for kidney stones, too.

Then the September, 1988, *Journal of the A.M.A.* reported a clinical improvement of 73 per cent of patients who were given 480 milliliters of cranberry juice a day for three weeks. *JAMA* advised doctors to seriously consider using this nifty food remedy as a more suitable alternative to standard drug therapy.

Finally, two scientists from Madaus-Murdock Pharmaceuticals presented a paper at the annual meeting of The American College of Nutrition in September, 1988, in New Orleans, demonstrating that *powdered* cranberry juice in gelatin capsule form worked more efficiently within the urinary tract than did either commercial cranberry juice cocktail or fresh frozen cranberries. It seems that the high sugar content in both of the latter tends to erode the berry's medical effectiveness.

A dosage of 2-4 capsules daily between meals is often prescribed for patients suffering from such urinary discomforts.

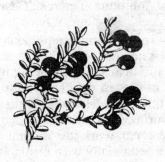

Dandelion

A great liver tonic

Several years ago I was an invited speaker at the Canadian Health Food Association's annual convention in Toronto. While wandering through the exhibit hall, I passed by one manufacturer's table which had a sign reading: "Try some of our dandelion coffee!" So I did, putting a teaspoonful of the dried root crystals in a paper cup of hot water.

I can say for all practical purposes that it *looked* like coffee, it *smelled* like coffee and, more important, it *tasted* like fresh-brewed coffee. This was my first introduction to a coffee alternative that won't play havoc with your liver (because of the oils) or with your nerves (due to the caffeine).

The fat we consume in our diets enters the gastrointestinal tract, where the liver secretes a yellowish brown or green fluid called bile that is then discharged into the *duodenum* where emulsification begins. Sometimes, though, if an undue amount of fat is consumed or if the liver isn't performing quite like it should, then not enough bile gets released to get the job done. The result can be a bad case of indigestion.

However, the same bitter components in dandelion root which give it that unique 'coffee' flavor and smell also manage to activate the liver into producing more bile. I recommend up to 4 capsules of dandelion root powder if you are having a meal that includes meat or greasy foods such as french fries. A warm cup of dandelion tea or, even better, dandelion root coffee, can work just as well. Or try 20 drops of the fluid extract twice daily with meals. It is also very valuable as a liver cleanser for alcoholics beginning recovery.

Lecithin is a term used by scientists to denote phosphorus fatty acids produced inside the body by the liver or found organically in nature. Lecithin helps in the metabolism of fats, so that they don't accumulate within the liver or heart, and it is also concentrated in the myelin sheaths of our nerves, protecting them from stress and infection.

Dr. James A. Duke, formerly with the USDA Agricultural Research Service in Beltsville, Maryland, pointed out in the January 19th, 1991, issue of *Science News* magazine that dandelion flowers have a lecithin concentration of 29,700 parts per million (ppm); soybeans, the traditional source, came in with a count between 15,000-25,000 ppm. One could just as well drink a glass of dandelion wine every day to get one's daily supply of lecithin instead of taking lecithin liquid or granules. I suggest half a wineglass (about 2 tablespoons) every morning before breakfast.

Better Night Vision

The February 16th, 1951, edition of a German medical journal entitled *Deutsche Medizinische Wochenschrift* featured an article concerning a remarkable herbal treatment for night blindness. A physician, Dr. S. Niedermeier, wrote about the value of dandelion flowers to help correct this disorder. But the substance in the flowers which does this, *helenin*, requires the presence of a certain amount of vitamin A. So Dr. Niedermeier devised a therapy program which included the dandelion flowers and fish-oil for correcting this problem, as well as improving the condition of a related disorder called *retinitis pigmentosa*.

It is recommended that fresh dandelion flowers (2 cups) be gathered by hand from an unsprayed field, rinsed in cold water, and then run through a juicer with one or two carrots. Spring is the best time for picking the flowers.

A well known and effective treatment for warts involves the milky latex from the stem of the dandelion. When a little of this is rubbed onto a wart several times each day, the wart will usually begin shriveling up and soon disappears altogether.

Dong Quai
Coping with PMS

After my trip to mainland China in the summer of 1980 with the American Medical Students' Association, I became converted to the health benefits of certain Chinese herbs, among them *dong quai* (also Americanized as *tang-kuei*). I contributed articles to the November, 1980, issues of *The Herbalist* and *New Health* magazines, appropriately entitled: "Tangkuei" and "Miracle Herb From China." Then again, in mid-1990, I wrote about this herb for the summer issue of a Canadian publication called *Country Health* in an article entitled: "Dong Quai: The Ultimate Women's Herb!"

Needless to say, I had been deeply impressed with what I discovered about this plant during our nearly month-long adventure in the People's Republic.

Part of the excursion took our group of 27 medical students and four physicians to the Shanghai Second Medical College in China's second largest city. We were presented with the case of a 27-year-old female college student who manifested the classic symptoms of premenstrual syndrome 'blues'. She suffered severely each month with bouts of crying, irritability, depression and occasional insomnia.

The doctor in charge had put her on a remarkably simple program which totally reversed these symptoms within a matter of days. Every morning and evening she would take about a dozen round pills — about the size of small ball bearings — with a glass of warm milk flavored with a powdered cinnamon. Never did we see the fluid extract of this herb being used all the time we were in China.

We were told later that the pills were a blend of dong quai and an, unspecified, medicinal mushroom. I remember noting at the time that mushrooms are rather high in zinc, which is interesting. An October 27, 1990, issue of *Science News* reported that studies had shown that women who sufferd from premenstrual syndrome 'blues' also suffer from a notable deficiency of zinc.

Another article in the July 20th, 1991, issue of the same periodical discussed the role of calcium in alleviating PMS mood swings and physical discomfort. This explains the purpose of the milk our Chinese patient was prescribed.

Dong quai itself contains respectable amounts of magnesium, and vitamins B-12 and E — all of which are important nutrients, specifically for the nervous system. No one ever satisfactorily explained to us the reason for adding powdered cinnamon to the milk the subject was given so I don't know if it was included for some, undisclosed, medical reasons or simply for its flavor. But I have to say that the combination proved very helpful to this young lady in getting rid of her PMS distress.

I recommend 2 capsules of dong quai *and* red clover and one 50 mg zinc tablet in the morning with a *warm* glass of milk flavored with a pinch of powdered cinnammon — the best form of flattery is imitation! Repeat the process in the evening, preferably on an empty stomach both times.

There are now more than 150 symptoms linked to PMS. Here's an easy workout to get rid of many of them. Sit on a carpeted floor with your feet together and knees bent close toward your chest. Rest both hands on top of your feet and place your index fingers at the base of the area between your first and second toes. Press that point firmly for one to two minutes. If you can't reach both toes, then do one foot at a time, and let the other knee drop momentarily.

Echinacea

Boosting the immune system

Remember when firewalking was all the rage a few years back? One well-known motivation hypester turned from selling used cars to persuading people to *think* C-O-O-L, and then having them *slowly* walk down a 20-foot-long bed of *live hot* coals to prove they could conquer their worst fears and tap into great personal power.

But I recall several ordeals by fire as practiced by 19th-century Native Americans which involved echinacea. According to Melvin R. Gilmore's 1919 treatise on *Uses of Plants by the Indians of the Missouri River Region:*

> "It was said that (Indian) jugglers bathed their hands and arms in the juice of this plant so that they could take out a piece of meat from a boiling kettle with the bare hand without suffering pain, to the wonderment of onlookers. A Winnebago Indian said he had often used the plant to make his mouth insensitive to heat, so that he could show off by taking a live coal into his mouth. Burns were bathed with the juice to give relief from the pain, and the plant was used in the steam bath to render the great heat endurable."

A lot of media attention has been given to *echinacea angustifolia*, particularly in health food and herb industry publications. But to me, as a scientist who knows his herbs, much of that is just old-fashioned marketing hype. If I were a gambling man (which I'm not), I'd lay you 10-to-1 odds on the other variety which you seldom hear much about: *echinacea purpurea*. That's where the smart money would be placed if this were a horse race.

Granted that both echinaceas can 'kick-start' exhausted

immune systems which might never finish a motorcross race otherwise. But starting something is one thing, and staying with it is another. *E. angustifolia* might rev up your lymph nodes a notch or two, but *E. purpurea* is guaranteed to remain with the action until the contest with infection is finally won.

Think of the immune system like your own private army, navy, air force, marine corps, and national and coast guards all rolled into one. That's how I described it in my latest release, *Double the Power of Your Immune System* (Prentice-Hall, 1991). This front-line defense system against infectious diseases is made up of your adenoids, tonsils, thymus, lymph nodes, spleen, Peyer's patches (on the small intestine), lymphatic vessels, appendix and bone marrow.

What *E. purpurea* does is to rearm these with the weapons they need for the battles of health ahead. The herb helps to sweep dead cells and other debris through the channels of the lymphatic system, and dispatches white blood cells to fight infection. It redoubles the power of the lymph nodes to filter broken-down material within the body. The production of lymphocytes and macrophages is escalated when *E. purpurea* is added to the system on a regular basis.

So how much echinacea should you be taking? First, read the bottle label carefully: If it doesn't say *E. purpurea*, find a brand that does. Then take 3 capsules every afternoon with lunch or between 11 a.m. and 1:30 p.m., when it seems to work the best. Figure on 15 drops of the fluid extract or a cup of the tea.

Evening Primrose Oil
Managing multiple sclerosis

A few years ago my younger brother, Joseph, worked as a volunteer guide on historic Temple Square here in Salt Lake City. He gave interested tourists the canned spiel of the pioneer history behind this and that other famous attraction, the Mormon Tabernacle Choir.

During his two-year stint he found considerable enjoyment in sharing with others something of his own religious heritage. That is, until he was unceremoniously and abruptly released one day for, he said, doing his job too well. This soon triggered in him rejection, despondency and a marginal desire for life.

Once his emotions had hit an all-time low, it wasn't long before his physical health also ended up in the basement. In the early stages he experienced restlessness, occasional insomnia, and what he described as 'darting pains' that moved around in his body. Later came infrequent muscle paralysis or temporary numbness that lasted no more than a couple of minutes at the most. These symptoms and some belabored breathing persisted. Two independent doctors diagnosed his condition as multiple sclerosis.

At the time his symptoms were occurring, I was doing extensive consulting work for a large Canadian supplement manufacturer. One of the better products was an evening primrose oil. I managed to bring a sufficient quantity of it across the border with me when I returned home. My brother started taking 3 capsules of this morning, noon and night — 9 capsules daily in all.

I also placed him on a ratio of 2:1 magnesium (2,000 mg) to calcium (1,000 mg); the B-complex vitamins inositol (400 mg) and choline (200 mg); potassium (2,000 mg); vitamin E

(400 I.U. to start with, then working his way up to 1,800 I.U.); liquid lecithin (1 tablespoon); and an essential amino-acids complex.

His recovery was slower than usual, because it took longer than expected to get his self-esteem, hope and enthusiasm back. In the first six weeks, the short periods of paralysis gradually ebbed away. A few more weeks later, those darting pains subsided considerably. In about 10 weeks his breathing became much easier, his sleep more secure, and his restlessness diminished by degrees. In three to four months his mind and heart bounced back and he became his usual jocular and likeable self once again.

I have never known evening primrose to work for MS in any other form than with the gel oil caps. Powder, tea or fluid extract just won't do in this particular case. The chief constituent in evening primrose oil, namely *gamma-linolenic acid* (GLA), has been reviewed in the clinical literature. Interested readers are advised to consult the following medical periodicals if they wish to learn more about GLA's effects on some of the symptoms common to MS: difficult and painful physical movements *(Lancet* 1:184-87, Jan. 26, 1985); hypertensive restlessness *(Lipids* 19:699:703; 20:573-77, Sept. 1984/Sept. 1985); other autoimmune and neurological dysfunctions *(Journal of Holistic Medicine* 3:118-39, 1981; and *Medical Hypotheses* 18:53-60, Sept. 1985).

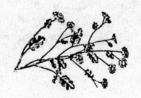

Eyebright

For better vision

British herbalists in the Middle Ages had a tendency to glamorize the benefits of this herb. Consider what Nicholas Culpepper had to say about it in *The Compleat Herbal:* " ... if the herb was but as much used as it is neglected it would spoil the spectacle makers' trade."

John Gerarde boasted in his own *Generall Historie of Plantes* (1633): "It is very much commended for the eyes. Being taken it selfe alone, or any way else, it preserves the sight ... "

But what can be soundly said about eyebright is this: if your eyes are inflamed due to an allergic reaction (hay fever caused by ragweed pollen, for instance) or bloodshot because of too little sleep or too much alcohol or infected with conjunctivitis, then this is the herb for you. A weak tea made from the dried or fresh herb is the best thing to bathe the eyes with several times each day.

However, capsules (3-6) can be taken internally for these same conditions. Eyebright contains an iridoid glycoside called *aucuboside* which exerts a definite strengthening effect on the capillaries of the eye. In the event your eyeballs aren't getting enough circulation, eyebright will correct that.

In the very early stages of glaucoma, it has been known to relieve intra-ocular pressure and to diminish shrinking of the optic nerve. The jury is still out, though, on its effect on cataracts.

Fennel

Death to dragon breath

The flavor of fennel varies greatly according to the type. Wild fennel is slightly bitter and has no anise or licorice-like flavor. Sweet (or Roman) fennel, on the other hand, lacks the bitterness and tastes strongly of anise.

In English cookery, fennel was well established before the Norman Conquest and was traditional with both fresh and salted fish. Fennel is still used with fish throughout much of Europe. It also goes especially well with pork, suckling pig and wild boar.

If you suffer from bad breath, fennel seed is for you. The quickest and easiest way to take it is to slowly chew a few seeds and let your saliva become sufficiently coated with its properties. Another way is to empty the contents of a single fennel capsule onto a small plate and mix it with an equal amount of baking soda. Wet your toothbrush and dip it into both powders, then brush your gums, teeth and tongue, You can also gargle with a tea made from the seeds. Repeat any of these procedures every few hours or on an 'as need' basis throughout the day.

The fluid extract can be used orally for the same purpose. Just saturate a cotton ball with some of the solution and rub it on your gums, teeth and tongue.

In England a broth or tea is made from 2 parts fennel seed and 4 parts barley for treating obesity. It is said that some modest slimming has been achieved by those willing to stay on this program for several months.

Feverfew

No headache tonight

Some of the medical literature published on feverfew in the last decade, has yielded some interesting facts. For one thing, said the British journal, *Lancet*, in its November 7th, 1981, issue, this plant can prevent blood clots from forming within the body. Another scientific periodical, the *Journal of Pharmacy & Pharmacology* (39:466, 1987) pointed out that "feverfew extracts are inhibitors of histamine release from mast cells." The editors of *The Pharmacological Basis of Therapeutics* (5th Ed.) cited internally produced histamine as being "implicated in the genesis of a variety of headaches." But if you take feverfew, then ...Voila! No more headaches.

Dr. Seymour Diamond's article, "Herbal Therapy for Migraine" in the July, 1987, issue of *Postgraduate Medicine* recounted several London studies in which migraine sufferers were given either feverfew leaves/tablets or a lookalike placebo. Those receiving feverfew reported the disappearances of their migraines, while "patients given a placebo experienced a significant increase in the frequency and severity of headaches ..."

The recommended intake is 3 capsules every four hours on an empty stomach for severe headaches and less than this for milder attacks. Or a warm cup of the tea or 15 drops under the tongue twice daily can be used. But I think that the capsules are the most sensible, convenient and easy to take, yielding satisfying results for even the worst migraine.

Garlic

Hypertension helper

Maurice Messegue is one of France's most respected and renowned folk healers and his patients include dignitaries from all over the world. Among his several books is *C'est la Nature qui a Raison* (Paris, 1972). Here is a true account from it.

There was one fine gentleman who used to visit my father once a year during the harvest season. He came from a distance, from a little village in the Pyrenees. He was the mayor. But my father used to address him as Monsieur le President to show his respect. I was also in enormous awe of him, first because he was such a big man and so ruddy, but also because he arrived by car, a luxury in those days, and came with Dr. Echernier, who was in his own right a person of great importance and my father's most illustrious acquaintance. Imagine — a doctor!

In view of the high status of these visitors my father used to tell my mother to prepare holiday fare — coq au vin, partridges and capons, foie gras and a number of desserts. I can still see our guest licking his lips over the foie gras, and sweating profusely as he gorged himself on all these good things. My father, too, would watch him stuff himself and when they came to the dessert would tell him respectfully but firmly: "Well, Monsieur le President, this is the last good meal you are going to have. Tomorrow you start on your diet."

For this glutton suffered from hypertension, which was the reason he came to consult my father. This last heavy meal had some of the ritual meaning of the last cigarette for a condemned criminal. From the next day on, this man was going to be restricted to one slice of veal with three cloves of garlic and three onions. Besides this, he would be allowed only some boiled vegetables, salads and fruits. He might also drink a few tisanes (barley water) that my father would prescribe.

Dr. Echernier was in charge of the patient and would keep my father abreast of his progress. After a month the news would be that he was getting better. His weight would be down and his blood pressure approaching normal. But as the months went on, he would begin to break the rules. And by the time the harvest season had rolled around again, there he was, potbellied and short of breath, come to consult my father. My father gave him the usual scolding, my mother prepared the usual last feast, and so on.

So it goes. If people did not overeat, heart disease would not be the scourge it is. But as things stand, it is the number one cause of death in prosperous countries. Abundance is a blessing, but we pay dearly for it.

Those suffering from high blood pressure would do well to take 3-4 capsules of garlic per day with their meals. Or 10-15 drops of the fluid extract morning and night. For colds and influenza, I've noticed that garlic works better at night just before retiring than at any other time of the day.

Because garlic is very hypoglycemic, however, those suffering from low blood sugar should carefully monitor their intake of garlic or onions.

I've just touched here on one tiny aspect of the power of garlic — one of the most potent herbs of all for all around good health. It is a fighter of cancer, heart disease, diabetes, and infections, among others. Read *The Miracle of Garlic and Vinegar* (Globe Special Library). There's an order form on pp. 98.

Ginger

Anti-nausea medicine

In the May-June period of 1990, myself, Dr. Earl Mindell (the pharmacist of *Vitamin Bible* fame), Dr. Morton Walker (the renowned podiatrist turned health author), and other scientists and businessmen from several different countries were invited to Japan on an all-expense paid trip as guests of the government and industry. It was one of the most exciting and educational sojourns I've ever made in my life.

We had a chance to familiarize ourselves with the local culture a bit, see plenty of rural and urban areas, meet with prominent dignitaries of every sort, and sample the varied cuisine to our stomachs' delight! One of the more interesting dishes served up along the way was a nifty little steak dinner using Kobe beef and ginger root. (Kobe is the place where they hand-massage the beef cattle every day to the background music of Brahms, Beethoven or Mozart, making the meat so tender you can cut with a dull fork!) Here's the recipe as I remember it.

Japanese Ginger Steak With Mushrooms

10 large dried shiitake
  mushrooms
¼ cup mushroom
  soaking liquid
1 tbs sesame oil
2 tbs safflower oil
¼ cup sake or
  Sapporo beer

1 tbs soy sauce
1 tbs ginger juice (grate fresh
  ginger and squeeze through
  cheesecloth)
1 tsp honey or molasses
1 tsp granulated kelp
2 lbs steak of your choice
  (Delmonicos will suffice)

First soak the mushrooms in a bowl of hot water for half an hour. Then remove when spongy, squeeze all of the liquid from them back into their soaking bowl, cut them into thirds, toss with sesame oil and lay aside.

Mix sake or beer, soy sauce, ginger juice, honey or molasses and kelp. Set aside.

Next, heat a skillet and add the safflower oil. Sear the steaks. Then cook them over medium heat for 3 minutes. Turn and repeat. When done, remove to a warm place.

Heat the skillet again and add the sake mixture, stirring to deglaze the pan. After 2 minutes add the mushrooms and cook for 1 minute over high heat. Remove pan from heat. Quickly slice the steak and arrange it on a platter. Pour the sauce over it and serve. Serves 4.

A colleague of mine, Dr. Daniel B. Mowrey, contributed a significant study on ginger to *The Lancet* medical journal (March 20, 1982) when he was still affiliated with the Department of Psychology at Brigham Young University in Provo, Utah. Entitled simply "Motion Sickness, Ginger, and Psychophysics," it demonstrated just how well the herb worked in cases of nausea.

In an experiment designed by him to test the effectiveness of ginger over dramamine (a common anti-nausea drug), 26 college students (50 percent male/50 percent female) between the ages of 18-20 were placed in a motor-driven revolving chair to induce motion sickness. The chair's rotational speed was varied between four and 17 rpm, with one of its legs being 6.5 centimeters longer than the other two to add a vertical dimension to the rotation.

None of the subjects receiving a placebo or dramamine was able to stay in the chair for the full six minutes of the test. On the other hand, those receiving ginger root capsules (2) remained for the entire time. And what was his conclusion from all of this? That ginger root "was superior to dimenhydrinate (dramamine) in reducing motion sickness."

Other studies done by him, and by me, have shown that

ginger root is also very good for the morning sickness of pregnancy and the nausea of premenstrual syndrome. Four capsules daily is the best way to take this herb. Half cupfuls of tea or a dozen drops of fluid extract beneath the tongue as needed also work, but not as efficiently as the capsules.

The *Journal of Ethnopharmacology* (Vol. 29) reported that researchers from Denmark's Odense University gave a woman who had suffered migraines for 16 years 500-600 mg of powdered ginger mixed with water when she felt a migraine coming on. Within 30 minutes, she told them, the migraine was stopped in its tracks. The woman took powdered ginger for the next few days, then switched to eating fresh, uncooked ginger daily. She reported fewer migraines than before and said those that did occur were "of much lower intensity."

The scientists theorized that the ginger was effective because of its anti-histamine and anti-inflammatory actions. Since ginger is not known to cause serious side-effects, they recommended powdered or fresh ginger to adult and juvenile migraine sufferers.

I decided to try both this and feverfew on one of our secretaries, who occasionally suffered from repeated headaches. She was instructed to take 2 capsules of each on an empty stomach with some lukewarm water. (The application of heat, for some strange reason, appears to expedite the activities of the pain-relieving constituents in both herbs.) About a week later, she was stricken with a headache while at home and followed my instructions. Within 10 minutes, she said, her headache was gone!

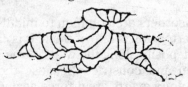

Ginkgo Biloba
Surprises from a prehistoric fossil

The maidenhair or ginkgo tree has probably existed on earth longer than any other tree now living — which is probably why Charles Darwin termed it "a living fossil."

The ginkgo tree is the sole surviving species of the group of plants known as *ginkgoales*, which go back more than 200 million years. They were around in the days of the dinosaurs! Apparently the group of trees to which the ginkgo belongs evolved from ancient seed ferns during Permian times. Trees of the genus have existed since the late Triassic or earliest Jurassic period.

During the Tertiary and Quaternary periods of our world's history, great upheavals of the earth, followed later by an ice age, destroyed the ginkgo trees and other ginkgoales in most of the world. The destruction was least severe in east Asia, and probably all of the ginkgo trees known today come from this part of the world.

It's doubtful, however, whether a natural stand of ginkgo trees is to be found anywhere in the world today. Fortunately for the trees, its recent history has been extended by man's appreciation of its beauty and usefulness as a shade tree and as a wonderful healing herb with many therapeutic applications.

Circulatory disorders are common to middle-aged and elderly folks. Hypertension is one of them. It is caused by cholesterol plaque deposits along the walls of the arteries, making them harden and constrict. Because the arteries are constricted, tle blood exerts great force against the walls of the blood vessels, causing the blood pressure to rise. Hardening of the arteries is another consequence because the arteries narrow due to these same fatty deposits.

A third circulatory disorder is Buerger's disease. Common to people who smoke, it is a chronic inflammation of the veins and arteries in the lower extremities. What's often referred to as a 'pins and needles' sensation is one of the symptoms. A fourth serious circulatory condition is called Raynaud's disease. This is marked by constriction and spasm of the blood vessels in the extremities, the fingers, toes and tip of the nose. This disease most commonly affects women and can lead to gangrene if left untreated. Additionally, poor circulation can result from varicose veins that develop because of a loss of elasticity in the walls of the veins.

A great deal of investigative work has been done in Europe on ginkgo and circulatory problems. An entire issue (September, 1986) of *La Presse Medicale*, a leading conservative French medical magazine, was devoted to this one herb alone. Of the two dozen or so reports published, about 25 percent dealt exclusively with ginkgo's ability to improve the memory through enhanced circulation. Another 15 percent covered different vascular problems, such as capillary fragility, easy bruising, and so forth. Individual reports dealt with improvements made in visual (retina) and hearing (deafness) disorders because of increased blood flow.

Ginkgo capsules can be taken alone or in combination (ginkgo/garlic) with other herbs. A nice program for maintenance purposes calls for 2 capsules each of ginkgo, cayenne pepper, ginger and ginseng (wild American/Korean combo) each day.

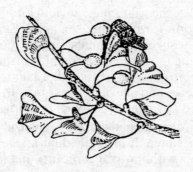

The Ginsengs

More than aphrodisiacs

There are three basic types of ginseng which dominate the world market of this particular herb. They are wild American ginseng, Korean ginseng and Siberian ginseng. While the first two are somewhat similar, they differ in some respects. The wild American is an endangered species in some states and consequently banned from being harvested.

It also has a different root configuration than the Oriental varieties. Because of this, it can command hundreds of dollars per pound — far more than the others. The Chinese seem to prefer our limited variety over the abundantly available Korean ginseng and many enthusiasts have been willing to pay tens of thousands of dollars for quite a small batch of the stuff.

Siberian ginseng is altogether different from the other two, both in function as well as appearance. It has a spiny stem and displays adaptogenic properties. This means that the properties of whatever else it is used with are maximized — they become more effective. For example, when used with antibiotic herbs such as garlic or goldenseal root, it increases their overall effectiveness.

For centuries, the wild American and Korean ginsengs have had a reputation for boosting sexuality. Evidence gathered in laboratory tests using animals tends to confirm this. Male rats fed ginseng mounted their female partners far more frequently. Siberian ginseng, on the other hand, has been shown to provide energy and alleviate stress in both animals and humans exposed to excessive sexual activities.

While it can't be claimed that someone will experience peak sexual performance, if an individual takes enough ginseng it can be said (without exaggeration) that they will be able to perform the act for a longer period of time before becoming exhausted. An average of 4 capsules containing a combination of both ginsengs (American and Korean) is suggested before such intimate actions begin. And up to 6 capsules of Siberian ginseng may be necessary afterwards.

A True Heal-All

A retired USDA plant scientist and a former Smithsonian botanist, James A. Duke and Edward S. Ayensu, believe that Korean ginseng is a true panacea for a wide variety of ailments. In their two-volume reference work, *Medicinal Plants of China* (1:123) they report that it is good for the following: insomnia, anemia, pain, eating disorders, asthma, bronchitis, hardening of the arteries, boils, bruises, cancer, heart problems, intestinal gas, convulsions, coughing, physical weakness, diabetes, gout, kidney disease, dysentery, dysmenorrhea, heartburn, epilepsy, fever, absent-mindedness, gastritis, alcoholic hangover and recovery from alcoholism, headache, bleeding hypertension and hypotension, nausea, nervousness, sores, dizziness and fear of heights.

Ginseng may be taken the following ways each day: 2 capsules; 1 cup of tea or liquid tonic; 15 drops of fluid extract under the tongue. It always works best on an empty stomach.

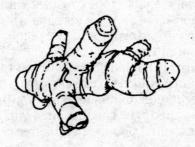

Glucomannan

Feeling full without filling up

Glucomannan or Konjac mannan is a *polysaccharide* obtained from the tubers of a perennial plant widely cultivated throughout the east from Indonesia to Japan. In such places it's employed in the preparation of a foodstuff known as konjaku flour. Processing of konjaku flour by one of several methods yields glucomannan.

The most remarkable thing about glucomannan is what happens when it comes into contact with liquid — it expands to 60 times its original volume when taken internally. This phenomenon has caused the product to be marketed as a weight loss aid in the belief that this increased bulk in the gut produces a sense of fullness. To some extent this is correct, but, in reality, glucomannan is a rather effective albeit somewhat slow bulk laxative.

A practical way in which to use this is with cereal grains. For example, one morning have two buckwheat pancakes for breakfast and another morning have two slices of seven-grain French toast, both with maple syrup. Around 11:00 a.m. or when hunger sets in, take four capsules with a full glass of water. By the time dinner arrives, consider whole-grain breads, rolls, or muffins or pastas or a baked potato (with the skin intact) for supper items.

You've effectively limited yourself to just two meals a day. Several smaller meals and two capsules every couple of hours may be another option to pursue. Whatever program is right for you, rest assured that glucomannan will definitely help you to shed unwanted pounds in a matter of weeks.

Goldenseal

Herbal hope for diabetes

A couple of years ago there was a run on goldenseal root in hundreds of health food stores around the country. It seems that someone told his best friend, who told his next-door neighbor, who told his uncle's cousin once removed, that taking this herb would clear the system of any traces of illicit drugs.

Immediately, a lot of young-to-middle-aged consumers made a mad dash for their nearest herb emporium to buy up what was in stock in order to pass drug tests of various kinds. But while retailers and manufacturers did a brisk business, the customers ultimately came out on the short end of things because I have to report, I'm afraid, that there just isn't any truth to that very widespread rumor at all!

But this herb is useful in a lot of other ways. It puts infections down, slows bleeding to a minimum, and its *berberine* content is one of the few chemical substances which can cross the blood-brain barrier (nicotine, caffeine, ethanol and cocaine being some of the others). Maybe this is why turn-of-the-century doctors used it in conjunction with red pepper to cure chronic alcoholism.

One thing is certain though. Goldenseal will bring elevated blood sugar levels plunging to the basement and step up the production of insulin in the pancreas. For adult-onset (Type II) diabetics this comes as great news, but for hypoglycemics it is something to watch most carefully. An average of two capsules twice daily with meals will help, but won't cure, the diabetes condition. The fluid extract (15 drops twice daily) is also good for this. The tea makes an ideal skin wash for eczema, psoriasis, hives and general rash.

Gotu Kola

The smart weed

This is an abundant weed growing throughout the tropical regions of the world. As a slender, creeping plant it is virtually impossible to domesticate in the common garden — but just throw some seeds on the ground, drive over them with your car, never water them, and generally neglect them and pretty soon the stuff will be growing everywhere!

The first week of September, 1984, found me at Airlangga University in Surabaya, Indonesia, delivering a paper on gotu kola to almost 700 delegates from 20 different countries. It was the 2nd International Congress for The Study of Traditional Asian Medicine which had convened for the purpose of discussing medicinal plants. And my presentation gave an old myth some new validity.

Some American and Canadian herbal companies have promoted this herb as 'brain food' to make you smarter. For a while I thought they were just perpetuating an old wives' tale. That was until I discovered two important clinical studies published in Indian medical literature by one Dr. M.V.R. Appa Rao. Then I had to revise some of my negative opinions about these claims.

In the *Journal of Research in Indian Medicine* (8(4):9-13, 1973), Dr. Rao discussed the benefits of *madookaparni* (the herb's Sanskrit name) in relation to improving the general Intelligence Quotient of mentally retarded children. Thirty boys and girls between the ages of seven and 18 were selected from a local school for the handicapped in the city of Madras to participate in the study.

Before the experiment began, all of the children were tested with a special psychological exam and their I.Q. duly recorded. They were then divided into two groups, one receiving gotu kola and the other a lookalike placebo. The herb group was given a single 500 mg tablet of gotu kola each day for a period of three months.

Careful records were kept of each group's behavioral patterns. Did the gotu kola work in those kids with mental capabilities of only a nine-year-old? Well, the data suggests it did. Some of the more amazing statistics are considered in the table below.

I.Q.s of Children in Study Group

Gotu Kola Group		Placebo Group	
Before	After	Before	After
17.70	28.41	26.60	28.04
43.60	54.10	37.50	38.09
37.00	46.50	39.30	43.27
41.60	53.06	33.30	35.37
33.30	43.54	38.00	38.60
33.00	47.15	19.80	21.54

To quote from Dr. Rao's report directly: "The overall general adjustment of certain children in the drug (gotu kola) group underwent a conspicuous change. Those children who were very shy and withdrawn and who were very restless and fidgety became expressive, communicative and cooperative, after drug administration (gotu kola therapy). The drug was also noted to have increased powers of concentration and attention."

Roa and his associates concluded by saying that "Mandookaparni (gotu kola) could be used for the routine treatment of mental retardation."

So how does one become 'smarter' or utilize his or her brain to its fullest capacity? Undoubtedly it would be helpful to take gotu kola on a consistent basis. Four capsules a day with meals is advisable. The tea or fluid extract may be all right for other things such as skin infections, for instance, but the capsules seem to be most ideal when it comes to sharpening the memory.

Hawthorn

Tonic for the heart

In medieval England the hawthorn was regarded as sacred, from an old tradition that suggested that from twigs of the hawthorn bush was fashioned the Crown of Thorns that Jesus wore on his way to the crucifixion.

Hawthorn blossom also delivers a dull, fetid smell which reminded many country villagers that it still bore the smell of the Great Plague of London. Because of this foul odor, certain carrion insects are attracted to the flowers and thus, in nature's way, fertilize them. These same insects usually lay their eggs and hatch out their larvae in decaying animal matter.

When I was in London in 1980, a middle-aged lady named Madge Vickers told me how she had cured herself of cardiac arrhythmias. (This is a loss of ryhthm indicating an irregularity of the heartbeat.) She said a doctor had referred her to an herbalist who prescribed a teaspoonful of hawthorn syrup daily.

"Pretty soon I started feeling better so I increased it to an even tablespoonful," she recalled. "Before long I was my old self again — no pain, no funny feeling inside."

While hawthorn obviously won't help every kind of heart problem, it may well be of therapeutic value for some. If the syrup is unavailable, then make a tea of the coarse, dried herb (2 cups daily) or else rely upon capsules (6 daily) to do the job for you.

Horsetail

Nature's beauty aid

Also called shavegrass, horsetail is recognizable by its erect, jointed, brittle and grooved stems which are devoid of leaves. The other layer of the stem contains so much silica (the material from which glass is made) that bunches of these stems have been sold for polishing metal and were once imported from the Netherlands for this very purpose.

It's also called 'scouring brush' in parts of Europe, and was once widely used by tinsmiths and cabinetmakers in England.

Going to the beauty parlor several times a week can be mighty expensive, but here are some tips about horsetail and other things which can be utilized for moderate cost in the privacy of your own home. Since silicon is so vital to the health of hair, skin and nails, it's important to always take some horsetail on a regular basis as part of a overall program for looking good.

The Hair: If your hair ends are split, have a rough feel, or generally lack luster, then add 3 capsules each of horsetail and alfalfa (for the calcium) to your daily supplement regimen. Brush the hair often with a genuine bristle brush — avoid using plastic brushes.

When washing your hair, make sure you use a mild shampoo. After rinsing once, pour ½-1 cup of beer over your head slowly and rub it into the scalp thoroughly. Follow this immediately with the contents of one large cracked egg and massage that in too. Then let both set in your hair for about two minutes, before thoroughly rinsing out with cold (not hot) water. The beer helps to clean the pores of the scalp at a much deeper level than soap ordinarily does, and the egg is for nourishing the hair with pure protein.

The Skin: Dry, rough skin that feels like sandpaper requires more oil and silicon. You should switch to a Mediterranean diet, which includes lots of olive oil, cheese, pasta, grapes, grains and so forth. In fact, it wouldn't hurt to take 1 teaspoonful of olive oil every morning before breakfast. Follow that with 2 capsules of horsetail and 800 I.U. of vitamin E.

On the other hand, excessively oily skin requires tannins and silicon in the body. The first can be obtained by drinking black or green teas or by taking 2 capsules of white oak bark each day. Three capsules of horsetail should also be consumed. And the skin should be frequently scrubbed with an oatmeal-based or pine tar soap. Then, after showering and wiping yourself dry, apply some tincture of witch hazel to such areas as the face and forehead to help close up the pores and decrease oily secretions.

The Nails: If your nails are brittle and break easily or have ridges or spots on them, then you need horsetail (3 capsules for the iron). In addition to this, you will also need some fluid extract of horsetail.

Apply a few drops, evenly covering the surface of each nail. Do one hand at a time and let the solution remain on for about five to seven minutes or until dried. Repeat the procedure on the other hand.

Nail Note

From my Chinese friend, Dr. Liu of Hong Kong, I present here some specific nail disorders which may reflect particular health problems, and the herbs, horsetail included, which taken daily might help each condition.

◉ Thick nails usually indicate poor blood circulation. For this you need horsetail (2 capsules), cayenne (2 capsules) and ginger (2 capsules).

◉ Lengthwise ridges sometimes means kidney dysfunction and anemia. For this you would require horsetail (2 capsules), buchu (2 capsules), dandelion (2 capsules) and parsley (2 capsules).

56

If the ridges tend to turn up and down, it's usually a sign of impending arthritis. For this you may need alfalfa (4-6 capsules) and yarrow (2-4 capsules), as well as horsetail (3 capsules).

● Deep blue nails might signify lung difficulties. For this you might need some warm horehound and coltsfoot (equal parts) tea (1 cup every four to six hours) and peppermint tea (1 cup). Horsetail (2 capsules) and goldenseal (1 capsule) should also be taken.

● Nails that peel, chip, crack or break quite frequently indicate bad digestion and poor food assimilation. Horsetail (3 capsules), alfalfa (4 capsules), dandelion (2 capsules) and peppermint (4 capsules) with any meal of your choice each day. Acidophilus may also be necessary to help improve digestion.

● Abnormally wide and nearly square nails may hint at a hormone imbalance in some women. In such instances, horsetail (2 capsules) and black cohosh (3 capsules) may help.

Horsetail is one of those herbs which I've discovered works well with just about any other herb.

With this marvelous little gem of a plant, you can really beautify yourself without paying a lot in the process. It's almost like having your own in-home beautician.

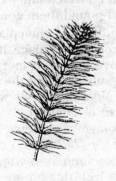

Juniper
Nature's disinfectant

Certain herbs and spices have always been used to flavor various liquors, beers, wines and liqueurs. Gin was originally developed in the late 1500s by a Dutch pharmacist from the extract of juniper berries in order to market a low-cost diuretic. It was subsequently adopted and popularized by the British, especially as a drink in colonies such as India.

My own personal experience with juniper happened about a decade ago on our family ranch in southern Utah near the popular tourist resort of Bryce Canyon. A hired ranch hand and I were attempting to fix a makeshift barbed wire gate when the palm of my right hand was accidentally lacerated by the rusty barbs.

I asked the ranch hand to go to a nearby juniper tree and pick as many of the berries as he could carry in one glove. Since there was no other form of disinfectant around, it had occurred to me, in a sudden flash of inspiration, that this would suffice instead. I asked him to put the berries inside a wet bandanna and pound them good with a hammer.

This primitive poultice was then placed directly on the injury itself and securely tied in place. It remained there overnight and was removed the next morning. By that time the swelling had nicely subsided and the nasty gash had neatly closed up by itself. Nothing further was done and I experienced no infection or discomfort.

Back in 1984, I remember reading in the science journal called *Phytochemistry* (23(6):1207) a little mention of juniper berry being good for *herpes simplex* sores. Well, when I was in Los Angeles lecturing for one of the Whole Life Expos, I referred to this matter in passing.

After my lecture was over and the usual crowd of a hundred or so people gathered around me outside the room for book autographs and many different health questions, one lady asked above the din, "Can this be used on bedsores?" To which I shouted back, "I can't see why not." She took one of my business cards and left.

About six weeks later a postcard came in the mail with a return address from Torrance, California. It was a short note of thanks from this grateful lady, in which she briefly explained how the fluid extract of juniper had helped her bedridden mother overcome infectious bedsores.

"I just keep putting the stuff on everyday with a Q-tip," she wrote, "and before I knew, just about all of Mom's sores were gone. Thanks for the advice."

Banishes Warts

Another time I was speaking at one of the annual Cancer Control Society symposiums at the Ambassador Hotel in Los Angeles. In my remarks I referred to a footnote item in the Feb. 1954 *Journal of the National Cancer Institute* (pp 988), which read in part: "The dried needles of *Juniperus sabina* and other junipers have long been used for the destruction of warts and other excrescences, and for condyloma acuminatum (anal or genital wart)."

Well, almost right away someone stood up and asked: "Do you think juniper could be used to get rid of some of my warts?" When I asked what kind and where he had them, he replied, "Plantar's, and they're on the bottoms of my feet and make walking very painful for me."

So I recommended that he put some drops of the fluid extract on the padded center of a bandage and then tape that directly over the wart itself, making sure to change it again the next day. Or he could empty the contents of a single capsule and mix the powdered juniper with just enough liquid to make a paste, which could then be rubbed on the site, and covered with a piece of gauze and taped.

I never received any written communication from him, but a year later found me back at the same place and convention for another speech. This time the same fellow took me aside before I spoke and refreshed my memory as to who he was. "Sit down over here," he offered. "I want to show you something." And with that he proceeded to remove his shoe and stocking and held up his foot for me to look at. "See," he said, wiggling his toes, "no more warts! Your remedy did the trick!"

A lady from Brownsville, Texas, cured herself of severe vaginitis or yeast infection, just by using juniper tea douche several times a day.

And how about the college kid from Minneapolis who was suffering from a bad case of athlete's foot? He had tried just about every kind of antibiotic the doctors and pharmacists had thrown at him, but with little or no results. I instructed him how to make a strong solution of juniper tea and to soak his feet in that every night for half-an-hour or so.

I never heard back from him, but I happen to know college kids pretty well, and they're usually more interested in cars, girls and sports than in remembering to say "thank you." But it worked, of that I'm certain, because I've personally used this on cases that were worse than his, with the most satisfactory results.

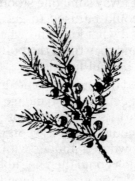

Kava Kava

From the South Seas

Kava kava is a tall, leafy shrub found throughout Oceania. Many South Sea Islanders, including the Polynesian people, use it for special occasions. The explorer Capt. James Cook first described it as an 'intoxicating pepper'. In Micronesia, a thick, bitter, non-alcoholic drink made from kava kava is heroically depicted as having 'a kick of a shot of whiskey with a Novocaine chaser' to boot.

My colleague and friend, Dr. James Duke (now retired from the USDA Germplasm Resources Lab in Maryland), described kava kava as being a kind of 'social sedative'. In other words, it relaxes you but still leaves your mind alert enough to capably perform all the necessary functions needed. To put it another way, it controls your work stress but certainly does not lower your job performance.

What makes this bush from the South Sea Island such a remarkable tranquilizer? According to the *Journal of Ethnopharmacology* (7:268, 1983) these sedative actions are primarily due to something called *pyrones*. In various tests, they have "been compared with the local anaesthetic effectiveness of cocaine," claimed the report. These pyrones "allay anxiety and reduce fatigue" without putting you under.

Kava kava differs considerably from alcohol in its relaxing effects. This herb doesn't impair your mental judgment in the least and leaves no untoward side-effects the next morning. It does not seem to affect work performance either. In a study of rats, scientists measured three variables, with and without kava kava:

1. Spontaneous motor activity — a kind of rat puttering-about that might be taken as a general sign of anxiety and tension; 2. The reflex action where the rat rights itself after

being turned over on its back; 3. The ability to balance on a rotating wooden rod.

Kava kava significantly decreased the puttering-about, but didn't affect either the rats' righting reflex or their ability to balance on the rotating rod. In other words, the kava kava left these rodents relaxed, but no less able to function.

While there are obviously many sources for kava kava, the best comes from either Samoa or Fiji. This is because plants from these two island groups possess the highest contents of those soothing pyrones.

A commercial pilot who flies for one of the big airlines told me at a health food exposition in Reno, Nevada, that he finds herbs like this have a very good effect on his mind and body. "When I fly that long Pacific run from San Francisco to Tokyo," he said, "herbs like this seem to calm my nerves by reducing my anxiety levels, but without numbing my mind." In such a profession as his, alertness is a top priority and kava kava seems to give him the best of both worlds — tranquility with mental clarity.

Because the herb is only available in this country in capsule form, no tea or fluid extract amounts can be given. The recommended intake for general nerve maintenance is 2 capsules per day on an empty stomach, but for stressful situations double or triple that amount may be necessary.

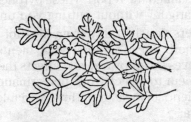

Kelp

Nourishment for glands

Kelp comes in all shapes and sizes. There are species which grow as much as 2 feet a day under ideal conditions. For our purposes here, though, we are dealing with *ascophyllum nodosum* which grows in abundance in the North Atlantic just below Greenland and between the Canadian Maritime Provinces (Newfoundland and Nova Scotia) and the British Isles. The icy-cold waters here are ideal for this olive green plant to flourish, as well as in the Norwegian Sea.

Norwegian kelp is especially rich in iodine, a mineral essential to thyroid health, vitamin E utilization, metabolic efficiency, and resistance to bacterial infection. The amount of iodine in sea kelp exceeds that found in land plants by as much as 20,000 percent!

The iodine from kelp has an affinity for the cells of the thyroid gland, where it concentrates and acts to disinfect the body's entire blood volume, which flows through this gland at the rate of about once every 17 minutes. Depletion of iodine results in fatigue, susceptibility to illness, inability to metabolize foods efficiently, weight gain and goiter. This element is also essential in the formation of *thyroxin*, a hormone which helps balance estrogen levels in the body. Besides causing weight gain, excessive estrogen is considered by many physicians and nutritionists to be a factor in the development of breast and uterine cancers. Iodine from kelp can be protective in this respect.

Norwegian kelp is also very rich in calcium. Kelp has always been a mainstay of the traditional Eskimo diet. In fact, the native diet contains five times the calcium found in the average American diet. Just one ounce of their local kelp, for instance, contains 273 mg of calcium, which is over 25 percent of the RDA (Recommended Daily Allowance). That kelp also supplies 25 mg of vitamin C when fresh, equivalent to the amount found in one fresh lime — that's about half of the RDA.

Another nutritional component of Norwegian kelp is *sodium alginate*. Studies conducted at McGill University in Montreal over a decade ago, and at the Harwell Research Unit in England, demonstrated that sodium alginate could absorb from 80-90 percent of the potentially deadly radioactive isotopes of Strontium 90 directly from the intestinal tract. Sodium alginate gradually chelates the remaining amount out of the bone structure into which the isotopes tend to become incorporated.

Nutritional Powerhouse

Norwegian kelp is an absolute nutritional powerhouse, containing many other essential trace elements. It has chromium, essential to glucose utilization; zinc for collagen strength and healthy skin; iron for 'tired' blood; potassium for healthy kidneys and normal blood pressure; copper for normal nerve transmissions; sulphur for preventing cell mutation that could lead to cancer; silver and tin required by those portions of the brain responsible for memory; silicon which is crucial to skin elasticity; magnesium for sound nerves; manganese for the sufficient release of insulin from the pancreas, and so on.

These many different nutrients found in Norwegian kelp seem to concentrate mainly in the glands of your endocrine system. They are scattered throughout the body and regulate many functions. Their chemical messengers, or hormones, travel throughout the bloodstream to all parts of the body.

Three of these endocrine glands are located in the brain. Kelp feeds them essential hard-to-get elements. The first of these glands, the hypothalamus, coordinates the activities of the nervous and endocrine systems from its control center atop the brain stem. A short stalk leads from the hypothalamus to the pituitary gland just below it, which regulates how much hormone the other glands release. And the tiny pineal gland acts as the body's clock, signaling the onset of maturation and regulating the menstrual cycle.

The functions of the thyroid have already been mentioned. But embedded deep within this gland are four tiny parathyroids, in charge of removing calcium from the bones and adding it to the blood. The bi-lobed thymus glands stimulate the production of white blood cells.

Perched atop each kidney are the adrenal glands. They influence metabolism, maintain normal blood pressure, and help the body adjust to stress. In between the kidneys is the pancreas which secretes insulin and glucagon to control the level of blood sugar within the body. The adrenals and pancreas, along with the liver, greatly contribute to the level of energy we have in our muscles at any given time. When our energy reservoirs are down and the body becomes fatigued, then kelp is called for. Certain rare trace minerals like boron, bromine, and zirconium, found in infinitesimal amounts in kelp, go to different receptor sites in each of these organs and help to chemically 'crank up' the body's energy supplies.

Finally, there are the reproductive organs which complete the last of the endocrine group. Male sex hormones are made in the testes of men and stimulate their sexual development. Women's ovaries secrete the hormones estrogren and progesterone, which enable them to safely bear children. Women who are thirtysomething and have been taking kelp regularly seem to have a far lower incidence of abnormal childbirths than do others who seldom or never use kelp.

Besides the numerous minerals and vitamins A, B-complex, C, E, D and K which it contains, Norwegian kelp is also abundantly rich in about 20 different amino acids. Some of these are essential: lysine, leucine, isoleucine, methionine, phenylalanine, threonine, valine and tryptophan. Without these amino acids on a daily basis, the body begins to die. The gut flora (stomach bacteria) provides low levels of them, but daily kelp will increase these levels.

Kelp likewise contains many conditionally essential amino acids. These may become important only under certain circumstances, such as inborn error of metabolism, infectious disease or excessive stress. For instance, one type of schizophrenic may have a recently expressed inborn error of metabolism that calls for more or less *serine*, while a burn victim might require an increase of amino acids. Certain cancers, such as melanomas, create tremendous depletions of phenylalanine and tyrosine. So kelp can meet all of these needs of *nonessential amino acids*.

Amino acids are converted inside the body in two different ways — either as a sugar called glycogenic or into fat called ketogenic. All amino acids, whether essential or not, are valuable energy sources which fuel our mental, emotional and physical activities. A lack of key amino acids is best evidenced in adrenal exhaustion and fatigue. But kelp (4 capsules), licorice root (4 capsules) and dandelion root (2 capsules) will keep our engines running nicely.

Salt Substitute

The use of powdered or granular kelp as a substitute for table salt has been gaining popularity within the last decade. Kelp has a pleasant taste and all of the necessary elements in a natural balance. Although sodium is present, it's nicely offset by potassium, which is totally absent from ordinary table salt.

I recommend that granulated kelp be used wherever table salt or black pepper would otherwise be used. This is a much healthier choice for your body's sake.

This type of seaweed also has a remarkable ability to stop bleeding. Simply sprinkle powdered kelp on the wound.

Licorice

Super without Superman

The licorice referred to here isn't the long, black rope of candy kids buy at the supermarket. It is a long, cylindrical, branched, flexible taproot, which is gathered in the spring and fall, cut into sections (1-4 feet long), and then semi-dried in the sun.

Of the 150-plus chemical compounds in this medicinal root, *glycyrrhizin* (or glycyrrhizinic acid) is the most active principle. Glycyrrhizin is 50 times sweeter than sucrose, and the addition of one pound of glycyrrhizin will double the sweetness of 100 pounds of white sugar.

But there's a downside to glycyrrhizin, which explains why Europeans use only the de-glycyrrhinized root, while Americans and Canadians continue using the kind with it still intact. The medical journal *Gut* (9:48, 1968) mentioned that glycyrrhizin causes "edema, heartburn, congestive cardiac failure and headaches." So, when purchasing licorice root, make sure it does not have glycyrrhizin in it!

Sitting atop the kidneys and pyramid-like in shape are the *adrenals*, the important survival glands. The combined weight of the pair varies from one-quarter to three-quarters of an ounce as the gland increases in size when stressed. Both physical and psychological stress stimulate the adrenals. The adrenal is composed of an inner core (medulla) and an outer shell (cortex).

The *medulla* primarily produces adrenalin and noradrenalin. Adrenalin, the survival hormone, accelerates heart rate and pours sugar into the bloodstream, which gives us energy and stamina. It raises the blood pressure and directs blood flow to the liver, brain and muscles during activity. In effect, it makes us super-smart and super-strong to deal with the sudden stresses being continually imnposed upon us by life.

But the adrenal glands often suffer from dietary and social abuses. They are constantly whipsawed by junk food, coffee, alcohol, overwork, insomnia, lack of exercise, anger and anxiety. This is what is known as 'adrenal exhaustion'. The most evident signs are fatigue, irritability, muscle weakness, inability to concentrate, indigestion, poor food assimilation and periodic bouts of depression. Hypoglycemia, or low blood sugar, manifests just about all of these symptoms, as does chronic fatigue syndrome.

Unless the adrenals are looked after, conditions can worsen and lead to serious illness such as Addison's Disease, which is life-threatening. Besides the more obvious changes, omitting refined, fried and deep-fried foods, soft drinks, coffee, and alcohol from the diet, and revising attitude and behavior, there is also herbal help. It comes in the form of deglycyrrhinized licorice root.

Licorice contains highly variable amounts of starch (between 2-20 percent) and natural sugars (between 3-14 percent), depending on the source. Both are quickly converted into energy within the body mainly through the liver and the adrenal glands. Licorice root is to the adrenals what a nice soaking in a tub of hot water followed up with a long Swedish massage is to tired, aching, muscles and joints. Licorice quickly tones the adrenals by relaxing and strengthening them to continue pumping out adrenalin but in more measured amounts.

Those suffering symptoms of adrenal exhaustion, hypoglycemia or chronic fatigue syndrome should take 4 capsules a day of licorice root accompanied by three capsules of dandelion root, or 20 drops and 10 drops respectively, of both fluid extracts. A nice brew can also be made using equal parts (1 tablespoon each) of both herbs in a quart of water (see instructions at the end of the book for making teas). Drink two cups a day with meals.

Licorice root also contributes to the overall strength of the body by aiding the digestive tract itself. Unhealthy conditions, such as ulcers, tend to limit the body's capacity to properly break down all ingested substances. As a result, the total assimilation of food and beverage nutrients is hindered.

The best-documented modern clinical use of licorice for the treatment of peptic ulcers has appeared in Chinese and Japanese medical journals. Patients are generally given daily doses of encapsulated or tableted powdered root for one or two weeks, with a 90 percent turnaround in their conditions. Licorice root is effective with duodenal ulcers, too. Daily doses of 2 capsules per meal are suggested.

A Utah National Guardsman, who served in the Desert Storm operation in the early part of 1991, told me that licorice root saw him through some pretty rough days when the conflict began. He said that whenever he knew emotional excitement would be running high, when his company would be engaging the enemy, he made sure he swallowed 6 licorice root capsules with a couple swigs of water from his canteen. He claimed that the root kept him from becoming fatigued, confused or overanxious.

With incredible testimonies like this, is it any wonder that licorice root can make you feel super without the caped Man of Steel beside you?

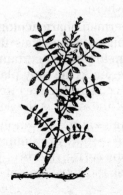

Milk Thistle

Protects against alcohol and drugs

On Monday, July 20th, 1987, I presented a scientific paper on milk thistle at the 28th annual meeting of the American Society of Pharmacognosy, on the campus of the University of Rhode Island in Kingston. The title of my report was, "Milk thistle seed as an effective drug therapy for liver diseases." What follows are excerpts from that paper.

Early on in man's history, thistles represented a curse on the earth — "Thorns and thistles shall it bring forth" (Genesis 3:18). Yet within the same curse was an implication of its usefulness — "... And thou shalt eat the herb of the field." All thistles are edible and quite beneficial for the liver.

Silbyum marianum (of which I speak here) is a member of the *Compositae* or Daisy family. It is closely related to other thistles, including common thistle. S. marianum, however, contains the liver protectant *silymarin*.

Though never mentioned in my original paper, I should point out here that certain substances can do great injury to the liver. The most notorious are alcohol and drugs of both the illicit kind and the over-the-counter variety dispensed at pharmacies everywhere.

The work of a German pharmacologist, G. Vogel, presents the most compelling evidence thus far of the definite efficacy of S. marianum in treating certain liver toxicities. Vogel noted: "In my experience the only plant product which has an anti-hepatoxic (i.e. a protective effect on the liver) action in the true sense of the word is the seed of the milk thistle.

"The seeds containing the flavanolignans silybin, silydianin and silychristin ... (but) are lumped together under the collective designation (of) silymarin ... We decided to test this substance ... against the most potent known liver poisons.

These are the amatoxins, phalloidient and amanitine, from the death-cap toadstool."

Dr. Vogel pointed out that the silymarin from the seeds prevented these three deadly compounds from entering liver cells, and when silymarin managed to reach these cells before the other poisons it was able to effectively displace or fragment them before any real damage could be done.

Toward the end of my paper, I cited a comment made by the California herbalist Christopher Hobbs: "It is fortunate that milk thistle has moved to this country and is becoming so abundant and widespread. With drug and alcohol abuse on the rise, and with the number of synthetic chemicals in our environment increasing, our livers are under more stress. As the number of milk thistles increase, we may be counting them as blessings, instead of cursing them."

Milk thistle seed works best in capsules or fluid extracts. A tea of the seeds can be made, but its effectiveness is somewhat diminished by heat. Since this is more of a therapeutic, rather than a preventive type of medicine, it should preferably be used when serious liver ailments prevail. Suggested intake is up to 6 capsules a day, given 3 at a time in the morning and again in the late afternoon on an empty stomach with some tomato or V-8 juice.

A 1952 Japanese medical study showed that tomato juice was terrific for regenerating liver growth! That's why I advise that milk thistle be taken with this type of juice. If you prefer, 15 drops under the tongue twice daily of the fluid extract can be used instead.

After I had finished reading my paper, I remember ad-libbing to my large and attentive audience: "Isn't it funny how ugly little weeds such as the thistle can turn out to be beautiful life-saving swans?"

Myrrh

Dental care made easy

Myrrh is the aromatic, gummy substance exuded by certain trees and shrubs growing in eastern Africa and Arabia. Ancient Egyptians burned it in their temples and used it for embalming their deceased pharaohs. It was an ingredient of their holy oil and a domestic perfume.

Myrrh was burned as incense for the sun god at Heliopolis at noontime. Persian Kings wore it in their crowns. Myrrh and frankincense were even burned during the reign of King George III of England. The gum makes good mucilage and the insoluble resin from the tincture can be used as a glue to bind parchments or book pages together.

A dentist friend of mine in Chicago told me that one of the most common problems in many of his younger patients is an inflammation of the gums due to bacterial plaque on adjacent teeth. He asked if there wasn't an herb he could recommend to his patients for this. I told him about the virtues of myrrh.

He had three of his female patients — all college co-eds — brush with myrrh according to the instructions I had left with him. They emptied the contents of a single capsule of powdered myrrh on a wet toothbrush (medium-soft bristle strength) and brushed their gums with it morning and night. In less than a week's time, he reported back to me later on, their gingivitis was gone for good!

Another problem dentists are seeing more of these days in their patients' mouths is *thrush*. This is an infection caused by yeast, *Candida albicans*, and appears as white spots which may peel to leave little ulcers. The breath is also offensive as a rule.

My dentist friend asked me about this as well. I told him

to have his patients brush with equal parts of powdered gold-enseal root and myrrh gum, and also to gargle with a solution of both, mixing the contents of a capsule of each into 6 fl. oz. of water.

One patient, Elaine K., had thrush so badly it was inhibiting her social life. He advised her to brush and flush with the mixture. In a week she came back to his office to inform him that her oral infection had disappeared. These are the kinds of results myrrh can achieve with dental problems.

One of his male patients, named Mario L., had a filling come out over the weekend when the dental office was closed. So he took some fluid extracts of garlic and myrrh and soaked a cotton ball thoroughly in the mixture. He placed it inside his mouth beside the aching tooth. In about half an hour the throbbing pain went away. He repeated this process as needed until my friend was able to see him on Monday morning. My friend told me about this and asked if I'd ever heard of these herbs stopping a toothache. I said I knew crushed raw garlic clove did, but not myrrh. Now we both know myrrh can do the same thing.

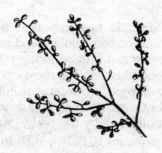

Nettle

Iron that won't rust

The stinging nettle is a perennial found all over the world. Its square, bristly stems with pointed leaves and downy undersides are unmistakable to the touch. These bristles act like a hypodermic, injecting an irritant substance under the skin when picked, so handle with extreme caution or wear gloves.

Interestingly enough, that same noxious substance is also discharged when a red ant bites you or a wasp stings you. Funny, isn't it, how vastly different forms of life in nature can share a common commodity?

Young iron-rich nettle tops, gathered when about a foot high, can be used as a spring green vegetable, usually in the form of puree, but their rather earthy flavor isn't liked by everyone.

In Scotland, nettles are combined with leeks or onions, broccoli or cabbage, and rice, boiled in a muslin bag and served with butter or gravy. I've had some of this myself, and boy, is it ever delicious! I've also tasted the nettle beer and nettle wine made by some folks in the Scandinavian countries. That is definitely an acquired taste.

Undoubtedly the single most important bodily function for iron is its production of hemoglobin, and oxygenation of red blood cells. It's the element found in the greatest amounts in our circulating blood plasmas. The most evident symptoms of iron deficiency are chronic fatigue, gray pallor and anemia. Diseases such as arthritis, cancer, candidiasis and herpes can severely impair its utilization by the body.

But according to James F. Balch, M.D., in his *Prescription for Nutritional Healing*, iron should never be taken in a multisupplement of any kind, only by itself. This is where user-friendly herbs like nettle come into the picture.

At a recent health convention in Los Angeles, a lady from Huntington Beach came up to me and asked, "I'm always so tired and exhausted, even when I get a good night's sleep. It just seems that my get-up-and-go done got-up-and-went sometime ago. My physician tells me I need more iron. What should I be taking for this?"

I recommended to her 3 capsules of nettle and 3 capsules of beet root a day — a capsule of each, morning, noon and night without fail, "This will bring your energy reserves back up there into the stratosphere," I said. "And won'w rust your insides either," I added with a wink and a grin.

Sometime after this, she sent me a check for one of my books, *Double the Power of Your Immune System.* Attached to the check was a gummed yellow piece of note paper on which had been scribbled: "I feel like a million bucks now."

Nutritional miracles like this keep happening all the time when people investigate the potential power of herbs. Nettle is one of those that have been neglected in times past, but it is now enjoying a revival around the country as more and more folks are discovering its tremendous iron-boosting potential along with beet root powder!

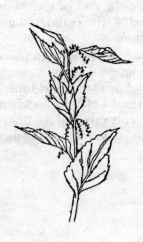

Pau D'Arco

Flushing body poisons

News item — (Freiburg, West Germany): The 36th Annual Congress of the Society for Medicinal Plant Research was held September 12-16 (1989).

Components of a remarkable Brazilian herb known as pau d' arco (Tabebuia species) were investigated for anti-tumor effects. Nine compounds were found to possess dose-dependent immuno-modulating effects on human immune system cells. This indicates that the ability of Tabebuia compounds to destroy cancer cells may be due at least partly to its power to stimulate our own immune systems.

A decade ago an Oregon man wrote me to say that he had given pau d'arco a 30-day trial after he was diagnosed with severe prostatis and doctors told him all the indications pointed to cancer of the colon and prostate area.

He brewed the herb in a strong mixture he called 'Taheebo Tea', using ½ to 1 tablespoons per cup, and drank 6 to 8 cups a day. At the end of the 30 days, he said, he was examined by a doctor who could find no traces of remaining bacteria or infection.

A high school senior serving as a nurse's aide at a hospital in Salt Lake City contracted a yeast infection. The girl's mother, who sells herbal products part-time, gave her daughter 6 capsules of myrrh and 4 of goldenseal until the candida went into remission. Twenty drops of the fluid extracts of both can also be used. This is also an excellent immune booster for AIDS sufferers.

Peppermint

Tummy treatment

The peppermint in current use throughout Europe and North America had its origins in eastern Asia several thousand years ago. Recent research has determined peppermint to be a multiple hybrid with a complex genetic makeup.

Centuries of cultivation have improved it, but also made it more sensitive. Left to grow in one place without transplanting, peppermint deteriorates and the leaves grow curly. It loses much of its flavor and aroma and begins to look like crisped or curly mint, a variant.

Fresh peppermint leaves picked and dried in the shade, transported to wide-mouthed gallon glass jars with tight-fitting lids and stored in a cool place, will retain their pleasant aroma almost indefinitely.

Years ago our family lived in Manti, Utah, where we grew our own peppermint. My father stored some in glass jars and we eventually transported it down to our cattle ranch in southern Utah and put it in a root cellar dug into the side of a hill. In the summer of 1991 I opened some of it out of curiosity. I was immediately greeted by a strong whiff of menthol. After all this time, the peppermint still held its flavor.

Taken after meals, either in tablet or tea form (I prefer the latter because it is a pleasant after-dinner hot drink as well as a tummy pleaser) it wonderfully smoothes the digestion, diffusing heartburn or flatulence.

The next time you go to your local chiropractor, ask him to place a few drops of peppermint oil along your spine from top to bottom and then rub it into the skin. If done before the adjustment, you'll be quite surprised at how relaxing it will be and even more delighted in just how easy the adjustment feels.

Psyllium
Lose weight fast

The way to think of psyllium seeds is 'good things come in small packages'. These seeds are so tiny that they resemble a flea in some ways. In fact the ancient Greek word 'psylla' meant flea — hence the name. Today, psyllium grows wild in southern Europe, North Africa and Asia where it's still known as flea-seed because of its small, glossy, dark-brown seeds. A hairy-stemmed variety native to India and Iran produces tiny blond seeds.

This is the stuff of which a famous commercial bulk laxative is made. By binding water in the intestines, psyllium husks increase the bulk and softness of intestinal matter. This increased bulk encourages the bowel's normal peristalsis or reflex activity, which pushes food through the colon. When food moves through the colon at a faster rate, toxins have less time to be absorbed by the body. Psyllium can also help lower harmful cholesterol.

An Italian study in the journal, *Pharmatherapeutica* (2:421, 1980) explained just how psyllium worked to help obese subjects lose a lot of weight in a very short period of time. Twenty-two obese women between the ages of 21 and 42 were either given psyllium or placed on a restricted diet. "The administration of the (psyllium) mucilage resulted in a weight loss greater than that obtained with diet alone," the report concluded. This was possible because psyllium swelled up within the gut, creating a feeling of fullness which resulted in a depression of appetite. Four to 6 psyllium capsules daily or 1 tablespoon of bulk powder in 12 fl. ounces of water should help a person to lose weight.

Red Clover

Epidemic control

AIDS (Acquired Immune Deficiency Syndrome) entered the American vocabulary over a decade ago, when doctors in San Francisco first began noticing a strange new malady that was killing dozens of young homosexual men with a terrible ferocity. Since then AIDS has raged out of control in this country and is now considered by the World Health Organization to be *the* single greatest epidemic now facing mankind worldwide.

Red clover is a common meadow grass, with a long proven history of fighting such menacing plagues as cancer. The following true account was taken from the *Phrenological Journal* of December, 1867, and discovered by me in the Sarah A. Cunningham Collection (fd. 7) at the Georgia Historical Society in Savannah, where I was lecturing on the immune system.

In 1866, Truman Woodford of West Hartford, Connecticut, after suffering for 29 years with a cancerous irritation that blinded his left eye and spread over his temple, wrote the following testimonial of his own personal experiences with this remarkable herb:

"During the summer of 1865, it had become so painful that I slept but little, was very weak and nervous, was confined to my bed most of the time, and expected soon to die; my friends thinking I could not live till the following spring.

In the month of August, 1865, I heard of a remarkable cure of a cancer by the use of a tea made from common red field clover. Thinking it was at least harmless, I used it as a common beverage, making it very strong, and also washed the eyeball with the same.

In less than two months, to my utter astonishment, the pain entirely ceased, and the sore began to heal at the inner corner of the eye. The healing process went on rapidly until the eye socket was healed over, forming a skin as smooth as that on my cheek, and the redness is now gone. The sore on the temple is also healed.

There is not over my eye even the semblance of a scar, and but a few scars remain on the temple. My sleep is now sweet, my appetite good, I am more fleshy than ever before, my general health was never better. And I think I have as few infirmities, and am as hale and hearty as any man of my age, which is now 80 years.

For epidemics such as AIDS or other cancers or some of the new kinds of sexually transmitted diseases, red clover tea is an excellent ally. Up to 8 cups or more a day, preferably on an empty stomach, is recommended. And when making the tea according to directions given at the back of this book, I advise using more rather than less of the dried, coarsely cut plant materials.

Red clover is effective in capsule form, too. An average of a dozen capsules, taken four at a time in between each meal, is very good. This and chaparral make, by far, the two best remedies against cancer that I know of. To this regimen can also be added goldenseal root and pau d'arco. The fluid extract works pretty well, but up to 20 drops four times a day under the tongue is required to be of any assistance.

Red Raspberry

Childbirth eased

The following information has been extracted from my book, *Heinerman's Encyclopedia of Fruits, Vegetables and Herbs*, with the kind permission of my publisher.

There are several basic differences between red and black raspberries. The red kind produces a spring and fall crop, with the latter being sweeter on account of the cooler weather (unless the spring is cool, too). The red raspberry has fewer seeds and is juicier than the black variety. The black is darker and its shape is odd, a skull cap rather than the ball shape of the red kind.

A Utah Mormon mother took raspberry leaf tea to make her deliveries easier. Other women in her local church and neighborhood often had more pain attending their labors than she did. She related that in the recovery room, after having delivered her ninth child, there were with her "several other young women who had just given birth also, moaning and groaning, but I felt all right."

She took a cup each day during her pregnancy. And just before entering the hospital she upped this amount to four cups of strong, hot raspberry leaf tea per day. Contractions started in just a matter of hours after she had been admitted; her husband managed to sneak her a large thermos of the hot tea, which she drank before being rolled into the delivery room. The doctor remarked that it was one of the easiest deliveries he had ever made.

Capsules can be used (up to 8 a day just before delivery commences). But warm water should be taken with them. The fluid extract is out of the question here. The most success I've seen has nearly always been with the tea.

Sarsaparilla

Clearer complexion

The sarsaparillas are mostly climbing or trailing perennial vines with prickly stems, short and thick rootstocks, and very long slender roots. The taste is mucilaginous and the deep orange-tinted roots are considered the best.

Sarsaparilla extracts have been extensively used as flavor components in some brands of root beer. Soapy compounds called *saponins* contribute to its foaming properties. Other food products in which they are used include frozen dairy desserts, candies and a few baked goods.

These same saponins have made the root valued as a wonderful blood purifier for several centuries. Some early-day patent medicine advertisements claimed it was good for many other ailments including syphilis, gonorrhea, warts, acne, hives and rash.

The saponins exert a deep cleansing action within the body in several different ways: they promote urination, encourage sweating, help expel mucus from the lungs and increase bowel movements. Probably no other herb is so thorough in cleaning out the body.

Up to 6 capsules daily on an empty stomach with adequate liquids (12 fl. ounces for every 3 capsules) is recommended. A tea (2 cups) can also be made. The fluid extract (20 drops twice daily) works well, too.

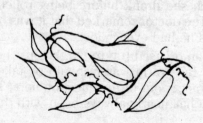

St John's Wort

Banishing the blues

This plant produces an abundance of bright yellow flowers by June the 24th, considered by many Catholics and members of various Eastern Orthodox faiths to be the birthday of John the Baptist — hence the name of Saint John's wort.

An olive oil-like extract of the fresh flowers acquires a reddish color after standing in the sunlight for several weeks at a time. This red pigment is called *hypericin*, which in very small doses produces a tonic and tranquilizing action in people, apparently by increasing capillary blood flow.

The 'Monday Blues' for many people, having to go back to work after a weekend of fun and relaxation, is pretty common these days. But something can be done about it to put a person in a better frame of mind.

A 30-plus lady named Cheryl L. from Smithtown, Long Island, New York, who works at a computer software firm as an office receptionist, used to have this problem — but no more. What's her secret for such a positive attitude and cheery disposition, while all of her other fellow employees still feel glum and moody on Monday?

It's the dynamic herb she takes in the little gelatin capsules every day that makes the difference, she swears. "I take two capsules of St. John's Wort in the morning with my breakfast, and another two in mid-afternoon if I need to. And I make sure I never drink coffee at night," she concluded. "This way, the caffeine doesn't drag me down." Ten drops of the fluid extract twice daily under the tongue may work, too. It's doubtful whether the tea can do this as well as the capsules or the drops.

Skullcap
Rubbing away bad cholesterol

My friend, Brigitte Mars, is a practicing herbalist and in-house adviser for Alfalfa's, a huge health food emporium in Boulder, Colorado. Like so many other herbalists, she had just considered this herb for its sedative actions, but never anything else beyond that.

Consider what she wrote recently in a nationally circulated health magazine about this herb: "In such a fast-paced world, we have a need for nerve-nourishing tonics ... (and) skullcap is considered one of the best tonics for the nervous system."

Now, Brigitte really knows her stuff about herbs and has been involved with them for many years, just as I've been. We have a mutual respect for each other, besides a general friendship. But when you're in touch with the scientific literature as much as I am, then you begin to discover things about herbs that go far beyond their established traditional uses. This happens to be the case with skullcap.

The work of Dr. Yoshiyuki Kimura is hardly known to herbalists outside the medical research community. His studies with skullcap, first at Kinki University in Osaka, and later at Ehime University in Ehime, Japan, have demonstrated something very remarkable in regard to liver cholesterol.

Writing in the *Chemical & Pharmaceutical Bulletin* (29:2308) in 1981, he reported that one species in particular (Scutellaria baicalensis) had a unique compound (skullcap-flavone II he called it) which "reduced the serum total cholesterol level and liver triglyceride content, and increased serum HDL (High Density Lipoproteins) or 'good' cholesterol." I've become a big fan of Dr. Kimura and have followed his work carefully for the last decade.

In more than one study he has presented evidence to support his claim that this particular herb is one of the very best (besides garlic and onion) for getting rid of the kind of cholesterol that can really foul up your arteries. This skullcap can also dramatically lower your triglyceride levels, which have recently been implicated even more as a contributor to heart disease.

In a 1982 paper published in the same journal (30:219-22), he made this concluding observation: "The results (of my research) suggest that (skullcap root) may be an effective crude drug for the treatment of hyperlipemia and fatty liver caused by ethanol."

What this means, plain and simple, is that this kind of skullcap can reduce abnormal amounts of fat in the circulating blood plasma which comes from eating too much fried and deep-fried foods, and can help reduce liver swelling caused by the excessive consumption of alcohol.

Up to 10 capsules a day of this skullcap may be necessary to turn around a sick liver; otherwise half the amount is sufficient for maintenance purposes on a daily basis. To my knowledge there is no fluid extract of this species currently available here. Where the crude herb material can be purchased, I recommend 1-2 cups a day. Either capsules or tea ought to be taken between meals for maximum effectiveness.

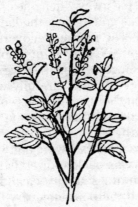

Slippery Elm

Lube job for joints and muscles

I quote the following four paragraphs from my book, *Heinerman's Encyclopedia of Fruits, Vegetables & Herbs* (Prentice-Hall/Simon & Schuster, 1988).

One of the most amazing accounts I've ever read concerning what an herb can do is found in the rare, out-of-print book, *The Woman of Mormondom* (New York, 1877) by Edward W. Tullidge. It relates in great detail how a woman named Amanda Smith was inspired with a divine cure, which kept her young son from being permanently crippled for life.

On Tuesday, October 30, 1838, the small Mormon settlement of Haun's Mill in Caldwell County, Missouri, was brutally attacked by a heavily armed band of religious hooligans. Close to two dozen young boys and teenage-to-adult men were murdered in cold blood and their bodies later dumped down a deep well for concealment.

Amanda Smith's youngest son had one hip joint completely blasted away when one cruel attacker put the muzzle of his gun against the lad's waist and deliberately fired. The mother recovered from her initial shock and prayed to God for inspiration. She was told by an unseen voice to make a lye out of the ashes of shagbark hickory, and carefully wash out all dirt and debris from the ugly, gaping wound.

Next, she proceeded to get some roots and inner bark from nearby slippery elm trees and pounded them with rocks until they were quite pulpy. This mucilage poultice was packed directly into the wound, which was then dressed with clean linen. The boy's mother changed the poultice every few days.

In about five weeks her son had completely recovered — a flexible gristle having grown in place of the missing joint and socket (which amazed physicians for years to come). The family later emigrated to Utah, where the boy enjoyed a full, active adult life without any physical hindrance whatsoever from his terrible childhood ordeal.

That's a true story that has remained with me since I first read it almost a quarter-of-a-century ago. I had always considered it to be more of a historical vignette than anything else. It never dawned on me that one day I might be drawing upon this account in order to actually help someone with similar hip socket problems.

A 69-year-old retired naval officer from Ventura, California, read one of my articles in a nationally circulated health magazine about slippery elm in which I related an abbreviated version of the Amanda Smith episode. He wrote to tell me that near the close of World War II, when he saw combat action in the Pacific theater, he sustained a serious wound when a Japanese sniper fired a single round into his body. The bullet passed through his left hip near the socket and exited. Doctors did what they could for him and his recovery was slow but complete at a stateside hospital.

While he was at first able to walk fairly normally, he said, over the years arthritis set in until finally, as he rather humorously put it, "Hell, I can't even dance a jig anymore!" He wanted to know if the slippery elm bark might do the same thing for him as it had done for "the Mormon kid mentioned in your story." I said maybe, but wouldn't guarantee the results. I told him to take 6 capsules of slippery elm a day for 45 days and report back to me. He did so and remarked, "While my left leg still acts up now and then, I'm able to dance with my wife again. That slippery elm stuff you told me to take sure is a lively little number, isn't it?"

A person can drink 2 cups of the tea each day instead of taking the capsules.

Uva Ursi

For bladder and kidney stones

This trailing green shrub has small leathery leaves that in some respects resemble tiny spatulas. Uva ursi is native to the temperate regions of the northern hemisphere (i.e., Europe, northern U.S., Canada and Asia) and Spain is the world's largest producer of the herb.

Jesus' injunction to the Pharisees seeking to condemn the adulteress he'd just forgiven may not be applicable here — "Let him who is without sin cast the first stone!" But in cases of bladder or kidney stones, by using uva ursi you should be able to cast out not just one but many stones.

There is an active component called *arbutin* found in the leaves, which is eventually converted to *hydroquinone*. This latter constituent not only disinfects the urinary tract, but acts as a small 'chemical hammer' of sorts to pound or break up hard stones, so that they can be easily eliminated from the body.

About 4 capsules daily between meals, or 1½ cups of tea or 10 drops under the tongue twice daily is recommended.

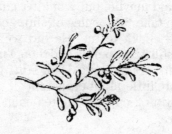

Valerian

Stress reliever

Common valerian is a perennial plant that is found all across the northern United States and into Canada, and it is also very common in Europe, where it has been the herbalists' stock-in-trade for hundreds of years. It grows to a height of 2-4 feet. The yellow-brown, tuberous rootstock produces a hollow, angular, furrowed stem with deeply dissected leaves, each of them bearing seven to 10 pairs of lance shaped little leaves. It is the dried, powdered rootstock that contains its marvelous properties.

Stress is always with us; we never can escape it completely. But valerian root will assist our bodies in becoming better adjusted to it. Its most active components are called *valepotriates*. These are like 'magic fingers' that chemically 'massage' our tight nerves just enough so that we don't go totally bonkers. Millions of people all over the world swear by it as a wonderful calmer. Its single most striking characteristic is its smell: It stinks like a pair of smelly socks or sweaty tennis shoes!

It is widely available from a number of herbal manufacturers at health stores throughout the country in capsule, liquid and powdered form. A tea is made by steeping 1½ tbs. of dried root in 1 pint of boiling water. Many people simply take a daily dose as part of their health regimen. For really bad stress, I suggest 5 capsules or 1¼ cups of warm tea or 20 drops under the tongue a day, or as needed.

Yarrow

For pain and inflammation

The many uses of yarrow in folk medicine date back to Achilles, who used the plant to treat the wounds of his soldiers. Yarrow has also been evaluated as a possible alternate source for rubber. And in ancient China, yarrow stalks were used by soothsayers for purposes of divination.

A locally published tabloid for senior citizens in Utah called *Golden Age Monthly* carried this interesting piece in its May 1991 edition, which I've summarized in my own words.

A grandfather had accompanied his married son's family into the mountains near Salt Lake City for a campout. On the second day his kindergarten-age grandson took sick with the flu. He developed chills and a fever and said his body ached all over.

The daughter-in-law moaned, "Well, there goes our vacation now that little Joey's sick. We'd better get him to a doctor soon."

But the grandpa spoke up, saying, "I saw a patch of yarrow on our way up here. Think I'll go get some and make some tea for him."

He put a big handful of yarrow in a pan of boiling water and brewed it up. His little grandson wasn't much for drinking the tea. He complained that it tasted "yucky!" So his grandfather hunted around a little more and discovered some mountain peppermint growing close by. He brewed some of it with the yarrow. The child reported that he liked it better that way. Soon he began sweating all over, but said he didn't feel cold anymore. Later that day he said he felt much better and by the third morning he was up and manifesting all of the exuberance and energy common to kids his age.

This is a true account of some white mice who overcame their laboratory-induced arthritis with extracts of yarrow blossoms. The arthritis symptoms, swelling and inflammation, disappeared within a matter of hours. As fully reported in the August 1969 *Journal of Pharmaceutical Sciences*, the scientists who conducted the tests attributed this success to the rather interesting 'protein-carbohydrate complex' within the flowers themselves.

You don't have to be a rat or mouse in order to enjoy the benefits of this wonderful herb. All you really need are aching, sore muscles, or stiff joints or back pain to try it out.

For relief of pain and inflammation, I advise 3 capsules each of yarrow and peppermint every four to five hours, or 1 cup of warm yarrow/peppermint tea blend every four hours, or 10 drops each of yarrow and peppermint under the tongue every three hours or so.

However you choose to use it, figure on doing so with peppermint accompanying it. For some unexplained reason that I haven't quite figured out as yet, yarrow always works better with peppermint than without it.

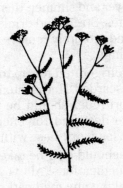

91

Teas & Extracts

The purpose of a tea is to extract the water-soluble goodness from medicinal plants. The relatively short exposure to heat in this method of preparation minimizes the loss of important but volatile components. The typical amounts to keep in mind are about 1 teaspoonful to 1 pint of *distilled, mineral or tonic water.* (Tap water is unacceptable because of pollutants.)

Use an enamel, porcelain, glass or stainless pot with a tight-fitting lid to minimize evaporation. Never use any kind of aluminum cookware for this purpose. Bear in mind that the tougher parts of a plant, such as the roots, wood, bark and seeds, require extra time with heat at a lower setting (simmering) for no more than three minutes as a rule. On the other hand, more delicate parts like flowers and leaves need no additional heat and should be steeped instead.

Once the water is boiling, add the coarsely cut, dried raw materials. If tough, cover and simmer, then remove from burner and steep 30 minutes. Strain and drink. If delicate, just stir with a spoon, cover and promptly remove from heat and steep the same length of time.

Most teas can be refrigerated for up to two days, but after this they should be discarded. Herbs intended for weight loss/cleansing and comfort/relief should be taken on an empty stomach, while those designed for energy/stamina and vitality/nutrition purposes work best with meals.

Caution: No herb should ever be taken with prescription or over-the-counter medications! Allow at least three to five hours to pass after taking any medication before taking any herbs.

To make a fluid extract, combine 4 fluid ounces of powdered or cut raw botanical with 1 pint of vodka, brandy, gin or rum. Shake daily, allowing the herbs to extract for about 15 days. Allow to settle and pour off the extract, straining out the powder through a fine cloth or filter.

Some herbalists insist that the best time to make a fluid extract is when there is a full moon in the sky at night. This, they say, enables the drawing power of the waxing moon to better extract all of the medicinal properties from such plants.

In the event you don't want such a strong alcohol base, dilute by 50 percent with distilled, spring or tonic water.

The amount of fluid extract per dose varies somewhat, but generally averages between 10-15 drops, placed under the tongue. It is diffused directly from there into the blood-stream very quickly.

One big disadvantage of fluid extracts is that the alcohol invariably destroys enzymes and some sensitive vitamins like B-complex and C, for instance. However, alcohol can draw out vital oils which water cannot.

Of all of the methods of preparation, I've always chosen gelatin capsules, for the simple reason that they are convenient to carry and easy to swallow.

Ailment/Herb Cross-Reference

absent-mindedness: ginsengs
Addison's disease: licorice
adrenal exhaustion: licorice
AIDS: chaparral, pau d'arco, red clover
alcoholism: dandelion, ginsengs, goldenseal, milk thistle
allergies: chamomile, ginger
anemia: ginsengs, nettle
arrhythmias: hawthorn
arthritis: alfalfa, chaparral, slippery elm, yarrow
asthma: butcher's broom
bad breath: fennel
bedsores: aloe vera, juniper
bladder disease: buchu
bladder stones: uva ursi
bleeding: (see hemorrhaging)
blood poisoning: chickweed
bloodshot eyes: eyebright
breast milk flow: blessed thistle
bronchitis: butcher's broom
bruises: ginsengs
burns: aloe vera
cancer: chaparral, ginsengs, red clover
candidiasis: pau d'arco
childbirth: red raspberry
cholesterol: alfalfa, dandelion, skullcap
chronic fatigue syndrome: licorice
circulation (poor): ginkgo
cold hands and feet: ginger, ginkgo
colitis: aloe vera
common cold: catnip, cayenne
constipation: cascara sagrada, psyllium
convulsions: ginsengs

coronary heart disease: chaparral, ginsengs, hawthorn
coughing: ginsengs
dental problems: myrrh
depression: St. John's wort
diabetes: ginsengs, goldenseal
diarrhea: black walnut
dislocations: peppermint oil
dizziness: ginsengs
drug abuse: milk thistle
drug addiction: ginsengs, goldenseal
dysentery: ginsengs
dysmenorrhea: black cohosh, ginsengs
eating disorders: ginsengs
eczema: goldenseal
epidemics: red clover
epilepsy: ginsengs
fatigue: ginsengs, kelp, licorice
fear: ginsengs
fever: catnip, ginsengs
forgetfulness: ginsengs
free radicals: chaparral
gangrene: alfalfa
gastritis: ginsengs
gingivitis: myrrh
glandular problems: kelp
gluttony: glucomannan
gonorrhea: sarsparilla
gout: ginsengs
hair problems: horsetail
hangover: ginsengs
headache: ginger, ginsengs, feverfew
heartburn: ginsengs
hemorrhaging: black cohosh, cayenne, ginsengs, kelp
hemorrhoids: aloe vera
high blood pressure: (see hypertension)
hip-and-joint problems: slippery elm
hives: goldenseal
hypertension: garlic, ginsengs

hypoglycemia: licorice
hypotension: ginsengs
immune system disorders: echinacea
indigestion: alfalfa
indigestion: peppermint
infections: echinacea
inflammation: chamomile, ginger, yarrow
influenza: catnip
insomnia,: catnip, chamomile, ginsengs
intestinal gas: ginsengs, peppermint
irritable bowel syndrome: aloe vera
kidney disease: ginsengs
kidney infection: buchu
kidney problems: butcher's broom
kidney stones: uva ursi
leg ulcer: alfalfa
liver problems: dandelion, milk thistle
low blood pressure: (see hypotension)
melancholia: black cohosh
memory loss: gotu kola
menorrhagia: black cohosh
menstrual problems: black cohosh
mental retardation: gotu kola
migraines: feverfew
morning sickness: ginger
motion sickness: ginger
multiple sclerosis: evening primrose
nail problems: horsetail
nausea: ginger, ginsengs
nervousness: alfalfa, catnip, dandelion, ginsengs, valerian
night blindness: dandelion
nutritional deficiencies: kelp
obesity: fennel, glucomannan, psyllium
osteoarthritis: alfalfa
pain: ginsengs, yarrow
peptic ulcers: licorice
premenstrual syndrome: dong quai, St. John's wort
prostatitis: buchu

psoriasis: goldenseal
rash: goldenseal
salt consumption: kelp
sexuality (repressed): ginsengs
sexually transmitted diseases: sarsaparilla
skin problems: horsetail, sarsaparilla
snakebite: butcher's broom
sore throat: bayberry
sores: ginsengs
stomach problems: peppermint
stress: kava kava, licorice, skullcap, valerian
syphilis: sarsaparilla
tetanus: juniper
thrush: myrrh
toothache: garlic, myrrh
urethra infection: buchu
urinary tract infection: cranberry
vaginitis: buchu, juniper
vertigo: ginsengs
vision (weak): eyebright
warts: dandelion, juniper, slippery elm
wrinkles: horsetail
yeast infection: pau d'arco
yellow jaundice: butcher's broom

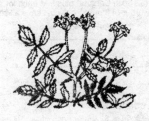

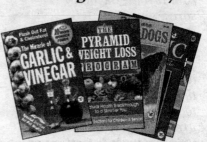